$\mathcal{B}$ODY ROLLING

BODY ROLLING

An
Experiential
Approach
to Complete
Muscle Release

YAMUNA ZAKE AND STEPHANIE GOLDEN

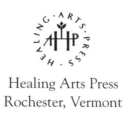

Healing Arts Press
Rochester, Vermont

Healing Arts Press
One Park Street
Rochester, Vermont 05767
www.InnerTraditions.com

Note to the reader: This book is intended as an informational guide. The approaches and techniques described herein are meant to supplement, and not to be a substitute for, professional medical care or treatment. They should not be used to treat a serious ailment without prior consultation with a qualified health care professional.

Library of Congress Cataloging-in-Publication Data

Zake, Yamuna, 1954–
Body rolling : an experiential approach to complete muscle release / Yamuna Zake and Stephanie Golden.
p.   cm.
Includes bibliographical references and index.
ISBN 0-89281-730-5 (alk. paper)
1. Massage.   I. Golden, Stephanie.   II. Title.
RM721.Z245 1997   97-22613
615.8'22—dc21   CIP

Printed and bound in the United States

10   9   8   7   6   5   4

Text design and layout by Virginia L. Scott
This book was typeset in Goudy with Snell Roundhand as the display initials
Photographs of Yamuna Zake, Susan Marchand, Patty Jordan, and Sandra Leatherford by Timothy A. Geaney

Healing Arts Press is a division of Inner Traditions International

CONTENTS

PART ONE

PRINCIPLES OF BODY ROLLING

ELONGATING MUSCLE, CREATING SPACE

When people come to a body-therapy professional with structural pain in their bodies, they usually expect that the practitioner will fix whatever is wrong and take the pain away. Many practitioners accept this role of "fixer," considering themselves to be in charge of getting rid of someone else's pain.

A more effective role for the body-therapy practitioner is that of educator. The practitioner as educator does not "do to" clients; she rather "does with," encouraging her clients to participate more consciously in their own healing processes. The key component of this approach is helping people understand not only what caused their pain, but also what they themselves can do to keep it from recurring. Once clients have this information, they can use it to heal themselves.

I believe that the body has its own intelligence, an inner memory of what it is to be "right." The body wants to correct itself, to let go of unproductive patterns of movement and posture, and it has an innate ability to do this. If you give the body information regarding possibilities for efficient and effortless use in rest and in movement, the body takes that information and uses it for self-healing.

This book presents Body Rolling, a therapeutic self-care practice for body-therapy practitioners and an educational tool used by body therapists to empower clients to develop a deeper and more subtle relationship with their own bodies. Body Rolling improves any type of body-oriented practice, from massage and physical therapy to bodywork, yoga teaching, fitness training, and somatic therapies such as Feldenkrais and Alexander technique. Developed through seventeen years of bodywork practice, Body Rolling is an experiential approach to learning the language of anatomy. It gives you—and enables you to give your clients—an understanding of muscle release based on internal sensory experience.

Body Rolling is practiced on a six- to ten-inch ball. While many people use balls in an improvisational way for stretching and bodywork, Body Rolling is practiced according to specific routines, in a sequence that follows the logic of the neuromuscular system. The general rule of Body Rolling is this: Muscles release from origin to insertion. Following this tenet, you place the ball at the point where a muscle begins, where its tendon touches bone. You release your body weight toward the ground via the ball, and then you wait and feel for change. The pressure from the ball begins to stimulate the tendon, bringing increased circulation to the area. As the tendon becomes more elastic, it releases from its attachment at the bone, initiating a release through the entire muscle. This release translates into a sensation that the body is sinking deeper into the ball, while the ball is actually moving toward the muscle insertion. Once you experience this change, you will have firsthand knowledge of exactly how a muscle lets go and what complete release really is. Then you can transfer that experience to your work with clients.

Body Rolling will help you maintain the health of your own neuromuscular and skeletal systems. In my years of teaching body-therapy professionals around the world, I have heard practitioners complain that they put out too much energy—they work too hard, they get exhausted, and their bodies hurt. Many are so busy helping other people that they don't take adequate care of themselves. Most body-therapy practitioners suffer from restrictions, discomfort, and injury as a direct result of their work—largely, in my experience, because most do not have a real relationship with their own bodies. Body Rolling helps you learn to listen to the useful information the body communicates to you, making it possible to develop greater control over your internal state and increase your ability to use your body more freely and intelligently, whether in your body-therapy practice, for exercise, or just in daily life.

This experiential basis is central to Body Rolling for one important reason—because the language of the body is not a linear language; it is instead a language based on sensation. Although this is unquestionably true, most approaches to bodywork training are conceptual, and so anatomy is taught through drawing, through book learning, or by building clay models of the body. Similarly, massage classes teach you how to perform specific techniques rather than how to experience muscle release. By contrast, Body Rolling is a valuable tool for teaching what I have come to call "touch-and-tell" anatomy. By practicing Body Rolling you learn to physically find the beginning of a muscle, sense from within what it feels like for that muscle to release, and feel the direction in which the muscle releases. Nobody *tells you* what is happening in your body; instead, you mentally focus your attention in a specific place in your body, and then you feel your muscles release through attention to sensation. Once this happens, you *know* what is happening in your body. And because the pressure of the ball keeps you mentally and physically conscious of the process as it occurs, the change imprints deeply in the neuromuscular system.

This self-work is essential to a body therapist's practice, for you can only impart what you know. You must experience the quality of the change created by increased muscle length, freedom, and mobility in your own body in order to convey this awareness to other people. The more you experience the nature of muscle release and the order and logic by which it happens, the more you can translate this awareness into your practice by first helping your clients understand why they have a given problem and then giving them a Body Rolling practice to use at home to maintain and build on the releases achieved in a session. As they work, your clients too will learn the language of the body and thereby become less dependent on you for information about their physical processes. Not only will your clients experience deeper muscle-tissue release, but their growing ability to perceive body sensations will fuel their curiosity about their own bodies. They can then use Body Rolling for further self-exploration, leading to greater body awareness and an overall sense of responsibility for their own well-being.

Though they give tactile information to others all day long, many practitioners do not teach the people they work with how to experience muscle release because the practitioners do not know how to do this themselves. They may teach the client a set of exercises for a specific problem, such as lower back pain, but those exercises do not provide the same experience the client had during the session. Body Rolling does. Furthermore, when you yourself have experienced what Body Rolling does for you, your enthusiasm will come through loud and clear, giving clients the incentive to do the routines you recommend.

One final reason why you should explore Body Rolling yourself is that there is not always a logical explanation for why certain releases happen—you simply must experience the types of connections that can occur. For example, a shoulder release may be linked to a release in the hip; or releasing the hip may release pain in the big toe; or releasing the sacrum may free up the neck and head. The more thoroughly you understand the many possible connections in your own body, the more astute you become in your approach to your clients. Body Rolling will enormously enhance your ability to pinpoint specific muscles and their connections to chains of other muscles. Your work becomes less mechanical; it becomes sharper and more anatomically detailed.

This book presents Body Rolling in a form that practitioners can use for themselves and with their clients. It explains the basic principles, gives guidelines for self-work and for working with clients, and provides routines for specific problem areas and common physical complaints. The chapters in parts 2 and 3 are technical in relation to the location and function of specific muscles. The muscles will be best located by reading these chapters in conjunction with an illustrated anatomy reference text. See the resource section for suggestions.

Who Can Benefit?

Body Rolling can be adapted to a great variety of clients; non-exercisers as well as exercise enthusiasts take to the ball easily. You can design specific programs for different needs. For example, after working on someone with sciatica, you will know which muscles are involved in that person's sciatica pattern and can give the client a ball routine that will work those particular muscles to maintain the longer resting length encouraged during your session.

People who work out vigorously can use Body Rolling to unwind and to elongate their muscles, thus helping avoid injuries. No matter how fit an athlete considers himself to be, due to the nature of his sport or the pattern with which he practices it, some part of the body overexerts. During this era of extreme cultural emphasis on physical fitness, people who have not been exercising with any regularity might suddenly begin a fitness program that includes aerobics, weights, running, or another high-impact exercise. But they almost certainly come to a quick halt due to injury, simply because they did not first take the time to feel and understand their own bodies. Body-therapy practitioners who treat structural problems know the importance of correcting postural patterns before training muscles; however, the practice of freeing up tight muscular holding patterns or correcting bad posture before beginning an exercise program is rare. Even if people begin with private trainers, in most cases the trainer does not evaluate body structure and adapt the exercise program to his client's needs. Yet, an exercise format that works well for one person can be an easy injury for another. Body Rolling enables you to say to clients, "Let's first correct your posture and educate you about what your body needs. Then you'll be ready to work out."

Whatever your pattern of tension is, it usually shapes everything you do. Thus, a massage therapist with extreme tension in the trapezius muscles due to overwork is likely to maintain that pattern while performing her fitness practice, whether yoga or weight training. Body Rolling will help her break such a pattern. It also works well for simply releasing tension from the day.

For people who hate the idea of exercise but feel they ought to exercise, or are told by a doctor that they must, Body Rolling creates an experience that is inviting (as opposed to one that feels like punishment). Even people who are overweight or badly out of shape find Body Rolling not only doable but enjoyable. These non-exercisers, many of whom may be uncomfortable about working with the body, will find Body Rolling ideal. It is exercise in a non-exercise form, one that combines the relaxing, pleasurable effects of massage with the toning effect of exercise. And because change is evident right from the start, they are motivated to keep doing it. After sitting all day at work, one half-hour of Body Rolling is more beneficial than a heavy session at the gym for relieving stress and tension, discomfort, or pain.

The Origins of Body Rolling

Body Rolling grew out of a therapy called Body Logic that I began creating nearly twenty years ago. Having practiced and taught yoga for over ten years, I knew a great deal about body movement and function. Then, in 1979, three days after my daughter was born, my left hip gave way; in the moment that it happened I heard the bones separate. After two months of trying orthopedics, chiropractic, acupuncture, and other healing systems, none of which stabilized my femur in the hip joint or relieved the shooting pains in my side, I got frustrated and decided to figure it out myself.

My theory was that the strong pressure on the pelvis during labor had caused microfiber tears in my adductors, making the left femur unstable in the acetabulum. Afterward, due to postpartum shock and exhaustion, these adductors temporarily lost their memory of function—only the hamstrings, iliotibial tract, and lateral quadriceps were keeping the leg stabilized. The most lateral muscles had become extremely tight to compensate for the weakness of the inner thigh. I started using specific yoga postures to release this tightness. Holding a pose, I worked with my hands to release the tightness, allowing the inner muscles to begin functioning again. Within ten days my leg was more stable in the joint.

This experience led me to begin working one-on-one with my yoga students to help them overcome their bodies' individual restrictions in performing postures. I began by placing people in a specific yoga posture, feeling for muscle restrictions, and using my hands to work those muscles into the stretch. I started at the muscle that originated the movement, moved to the muscle the first one fed into, and then moved to the next, continuing on through the line of muscles involved in the stretch, working to give each muscle its greatest length.

Soon people began coming to me with physical problems and injuries; of necessity, I began formal study of anatomy and physiology. As people came with more specific problems, I narrowed my focus from yoga to particular body complaints. And since I wanted to help in the fastest, most direct way, my work moved away from yoga into a practice in which I worked on the floor with the client lying over a pillow. With one hand creating traction, I used my elbow to work the point of origin of each muscle.

Over the years, in addition to working with everyday tension, postural problems, strains, and sprains, I have treated people with herniated discs; vertebral subluxations; shoulder, knee, and ankle injuries; multiple sclerosis; epileptic seizures; strokes; migraines; cerebral palsy; scoliosis; arthritis; vertigo; paralyses; sciatica; sports-related injuries, such as tennis elbow; and structural problems. I have also assisted people in postsurgical rehabilitation. All this time my work remained true to the basic principle of hatha yoga: to remove all physical restrictions so that energy can flow unobstructed through the body.

Body Logic works according to the body's natural logic and order: Wherever one muscle ends, another begins. Thus, its fundamental philosophy is to address a complaint in the context of the entire body, recognizing how the client has compensated for it and where that compensation begins in the tendino-muscular system, and then working systematically through the connecting muscle groups. There is always a relationship between the muscles above and below a problem area—a knee problem, for example, will affect the foot, the hip, or both. The key to repatterning is to see the muscles as a connecting chain and to release all of them, from hip to knee to foot.

Because many body-therapy practitioners are used to simply spot-treating the muscles in a problem area, they do not realize to what benefit they can use the fact that chains of muscles are linked. The key point for releasing pain in a given area is often in another area that is part of the same chain. One way to learn these connections is to work with the ball.

Creating Space

A unique aspect of Body Logic is its use of traction—both directly and with joint rotation—to lengthen a muscle before working on it. The moment you exert traction you tell the muscle what direction it will release in and give it freedom to elongate. Traction also creates intra-articular space, and creating space is the basic principle of Body Logic.

When a person experiences pain or discomfort due to sprain, muscle spasm, or nerve impingement, there is compression or restriction in a specific area of the body. In general, wherever there is restriction, compression, contraction, tightness, inflammation, atrophy, or nerve pain, there will be lack of space. This lack will first manifest as muscle tightness, as when a person cannot turn or bend as much as he could before. If this problem is not corrected, it moves to the next level—the muscles become so tight that they impinge on nerve, as in sciatica or numbness in the fingers or toes. The first step in healing nerve impingement is to restore length to the involved muscles. Once the muscles have their length back they stop pressing into and irritating nerve tissue.

Different bodies lack space for different reasons. People who do not use certain muscles over a long period of time, such as obese persons and the elderly, often have a collapsed skeletal structure. When an entire muscle is not worked over a period of time, it begins to lose function at both ends. As function is lost, the muscle collapses or atrophies, no longer taking its full space. The goal, then, is to create as much space as possible in the collapsed area by enabling the muscles to elongate to their maximum possible resting length while still maintaining vitality and balanced tone.

Dedicated athletes lack space in joints and muscles for different reasons. For example, weightlifters working to bulk up their muscles may focus only on the body of the muscle because it is the part they can see; they do not work the tendon. As they keep bulking the muscle, it shortens, putting stress on the tendons and joints. Most muscle injuries are actually tendon strains; most people do not realize that the muscle is much longer than the part of it they can feel. Muscles that do not take their full length make joints tighter because they pull the bones together. Increased bulk in muscle body without an increase in length leads to tendonitis, microfiber tendon tears, and restricted joint movement.

The concept of Body Logic, then, is to work the entire muscle, restoring its function at the origin. Elongating the muscle also creates mobility in the joint. Consequently, if there is tendonitis in the knee, for example, you look at what muscles have their insertions in the knee (which means they have their origins on the pelvis or femur) and what muscles have their origins at the knee and insertions at the ankle and foot. Then, using traction, you work the leg systematically to release each muscle from origin to insertion, giving the muscles their length from the hip down into the knee, then working the origins from the knee down to the insertions in the ankle and foot.

The principle of creating space offers a simple way to evaluate a client's body. The assessment technique discussed in the next section will enable you to determine which areas need more space and which muscles need to be lengthened. You can then consider what effects shortness in those muscles might be having on specific joints and go on to figure out what movements are restricted in those joints and what other muscles might have become shortened because of shortness in the first group of muscles. Using this logical process, you begin to see how chains of muscle can be involved in a lack of space you have observed in a given area of the body. Then, working with the natural order of muscle release, you can create the necessary space.

Assessment Technique

To train your vision to assess someone's body, start by observing the whole person. Body-therapy practitioners are trained to visually assess various body parts. But most important is to evaluate first what general signals a person is sending through her body. Ask yourself: If you had only one session to help her, what would be the one thing you could do that would affect her most profoundly? To do this, observe first where the breath reaches in her body. Does she breathe into the back of her rib cage, into the front, or into the sides? Breathing patterns are the most reliable indicators of restrictions. Thus, observing the breath is the quickest, most effective way to identify a client's core problem.

Another whole-body observation involves noting the relationship of the limbs to the torso. Are the arms and legs retracted into the center of the body? Are they loose in their joints and unconnected to the body?

Now you can start the part-by-part assessment. Depending on which patterns you see, you can determine which muscles lack space and therefore need to be released.

Look first at the position of the head in relation to the shoulders. Does it project forward or backward? Does it tilt to one side or the other? Is it rotated to one side or the other?

Next observe the shoulders. Is one shoulder higher than the other? Are one or both shoulders rotated anteriorly or posteriorly? Are they pulled up toward the ears?

Look at the hips. Is one hip higher than the other? Is one hip or both hips rotated anteriorly? Is there adequate length between pelvis and rib cage? This indicates whether the abdominal muscles are lengthened, toned, and supporting the center of the body in balance with the muscles of the back. Is the upper body collapsing, exerting pressure down into the pelvis and shortening the abdominal muscles? Are these muscles protruding or contracted inward? Does the downward pull of the upper body restrict leg movement at the hip?

Next, observe knee alignment. Are the muscles that insert on the knee balanced laterally and medially? Observe the position of the patellas. Are they elevated, dropped, or rotated laterally or medially?

Observe the ankles. Is the weight distributed equally on the malleoli? If not, are the ankles prolapsed medially, or is there tension and rigidity on the outside of the foot?

Finally, notice how the feet connect with the ground. Does the weight drop heavily into the earth, or is the person light on her feet, with a lifting quality in the body? This will tell you whether in general there is a downward pull on her entire musculature. Is there a lifting quality on one side of the body and a dropping on the other? This imbalance between tighter muscles on one side and more elastic muscles on the other can create a potential for injuries.

How Body Rolling Reeducates the Muscles

In developing Body Rolling, I took the principle of creating space and began working with the ball to invent a system in which people could do for themselves what we accomplished together when I worked on them in a Body Logic session. The uniqueness of Body Rolling is in the way it educates each muscle to release and take its optimal space. Each muscle has a natural memory of its function, a self-recognition that is programmed into the brain; oftentimes, due to habitual bad posture, accidents, or other causes, this program is altered. For example, cutting through a muscle during surgery severs the neuromuscular impulses that direct that muscle's function. However, the memory is still there and can be awakened.

What Body Logic and Body Rolling do as therapies is reeducate the muscle, restoring original muscle memory. The key to restoring this memory is learning to wait and listen, trusting that the muscle intrinsically knows what to do. In essence, all you are doing is applying pressure with the ball at the point of origin and simply waiting there until you feel the muscle respond. Stimulating muscle at the origin elongates the muscle fibers toward their insertion point, indicating to the muscle that there is greater space for it to expand into. The communication to the muscle happens via sensation; by waiting you give the muscle time to receive information from the brain about what its action is supposed to be. The body understands the physical sensation. The muscle memory reawakens, and the muscle regains its function.

For example, the deep muscles of the back work upward in an intricate interlayered chain, from the base of the spine to the cranium. If you simply lie back over a ball placed beneath the midthoracic area, as people often do to open up the chest, the pressure is felt in just that one area. The muscle fibers of this chain below and above this point get pulled toward it; they do not receive information to release. However, if you begin at the base of the spine and move upward, you build a momentum that creates a connected and continuing release of all these deep spinal muscles.

Similarly, if you just poke at or knead a muscle, as in some types of massage, you do not "tell" the muscle anything about function and full release. Thus, when the neck is tight, massaging the back of the neck alone will not resolve the problem. Moving the ball up along the entire length of the neck all the way to the cranium, however, lengthens the muscles that attach to the spine and stimulates them to release. Body Rolling gives people the experience of a completely released muscle, one that has its full length and tone and function all the way from origin to insertion.

Changing the Quality of Bone

Bodyworkers like to get their hands on muscle because it is pliable and you can feel its quality changing as you work. People tend to think of bone, on the other hand, as a hard, solid mass that is immovable unless stimulated by muscle. However, when you begin touching bone you soon sense that its quality changes under pressure. Bone has much more life in it than you might think—bone is living tissue with its own blood supply and circulation. Where there is life, there is movement, by which I mean cellular activity. And the more alive bone is, the more resilient it becomes.

Understanding the anatomical and physiological function of bone, you can focus on creating this type of inner movement within bone tissue. A bone that has arrested movement is dense; the aging process renders it increasingly ossified, and it initially feels quite brittle. But if you apply some pressure with the ball, the function of the bone begins to wake up. To me, bone is like dried fruit. Just as a raisin plumps up after you put it in water, when bone is stimulated and becomes alive it undergoes a subtle change, acquiring a supple quality that makes it seem more of a living unit with its tendon.

Most bodyworkers, however, do not work on bone. Although their work may result in some improvement in muscle, if bone is not stimulated there will not be a complete release of any muscle, since the part of the tendon that attaches to bone has not received stimulation. The tendon is the uniting tissue between muscle and bone—the more rigid bone gets, the more contracted the tendons that attach to it become, and consequently the muscle shortens and loses its elasticity, eventually becoming atrophied. In order to change the quality of tendon, you must change the quality of its attachment to bone as well as to muscle.

A basic Body Logic principle is that applying gentle direct pressure on bone will initiate release of the tendons of all muscles that have attachments anywhere else on that bone. Release of the tendons will in turn release the muscles. Therefore, Body Rolling always begins with bone. Studies have found that electrical stimulation of the tendon and its insertion in bone will promote healing of tendonitis and microfiber tears.* Body Rolling works on this same principle, with the ball providing the stimulation. When you place the ball at the origin point, then sit and wait, the circulation to the tendon increases. It begins to move and change in quality; the muscle elongates,

---

* Examples include J. A. Burne and O. C. Lippold, "Reflex Inhibition Following Electrical Stimulation over Muscle Tendons in Man," *Brain* 119 (Pt. 4):1107-14, August 1996, and J. P. Nessler and D. P. Mass, "Direct-Current Electrical Stimulation of Tendon Healing in Vitro," *Clinical Orthopedics* 217:303-12, April 1987. Robert O. Becker and Gary Selden, *The Body Electric: Electromagnetism and the Foundation of Life* (New York: Morrow, 1985), describe how muscle fiber can be healed by electrical stimulation of tendon.

and its movement becomes more complete. Working on bone in this way is what actually releases muscle.

Throughout the routines in the following chapters, I will be describing how to place the ball at specific origin points and work specific muscles toward their insertion. When muscles begin to release, the mind, perceiving that sensation, becomes actively involved in the process, creating a deep and knowing relationship with the body.

2

Developing a
Relationship
with Your Body

For the most part, people become body-therapy practitioners for one of three reasons—either they have been greatly affected by a bodywork experience, or they have been told they have "good hands," or they practice some kind of body discipline and have a keen kinesthetic awareness of the body. Those who enter the body-therapy profession for the first two reasons generally seek a program that will teach them a technique so they can get licensure to do hands-on bodywork. Those who enter the profession because of their personal experience with and attunement to the body process are usually attracted to a form of therapy in which they can use their own bodies as learning tools.

Both types of practitioners share a deep desire to help and care for others. Frequently they become so involved in taking care of other people that they do not take enough care of themselves, thus sabotaging their own skills and health. The work positions body-therapy practitioners most often assume become so embedded in the body that these work patterns turn into their habitual postures, because they do not take time at the end of the day to undo the effects of their work postures on the body.

At first these patterns do not hurt; the pleasure of helping others is so strong that practitioners do not even notice the patterns developing. Soon, however, the body begins to give warning messages, but without a method of self-study it is difficult to recognize what these messages are conveying and what to do about them. The work pattern eventually becomes a pain pattern that the practitioner lives with daily.

While practitioners are busy ministering to other people, they turn off their bodies' messages in order to get through the day, assuming that doing so will make no difference to their clients. However, when I teach body-therapy practitioners, I use an exercise to demonstrate that this is not the case. Requesting a volunteer who is in pain from his or her work, I have another student lie down on the table with eyes closed and ask the person in pain to work on the other. In less than one minute the one lying down can tell exactly where the other person's pain is located.

A body therapist transmits in his work whatever pain and suffering he may be experiencing. Attempting to push through pain will diminish the therapist's effectiveness.

Practitioners need to understand that bodies have their own sense of knowing. Everyone you work on has an extraordinary level of perception, whether they are consciously in touch with it or not, and anything you are feeling can be transmitted to another body. If you see yourself as a "fixer," you separate your own being from your mechanical manipulation of another body and you do not perceive that your own suffering is being communicated. When you become aware of the depth and power of touch you realize that you are transmitting your own pain, which of course is contrary to your intention.

On the other hand, when you are truly committed to your own well-being, you will transmit this attitude to the other person, on a cellular level, through your touch. When you maintain a stance of respect and integrity toward your own body, it will manifest in the effect you have on clients. We owe it to the people we help to take the time to take care of ourselves and explore our own processes. Through such explorations the body therapist develops a relationship with her body, cultivating a form of self-awareness that integrates mental, physical, and emotional perception. This integrated awareness is transmitted through the therapist's physical work on people's bodies, but affects them on other levels as well. A therapist so committed to personal well-being necessarily transforms from a "fixer" into an educator.

Most body-therapy practitioners say they do not have time for themselves, but the truth is that you need to set an example for your clients. If you are trashing your own body, you are not a very good example. It is true that developing a relationship with your body requires time for exploration and communication. Yet, if you will not give yourself this time, you cannot convince clients that they need to develop a similarly rich relationship with their own bodies.

In their struggle to be respected and accepted by the medical community, many massage therapy systems put much effort into describing their work according to the medical model and diagnosing and treating specific conditions. As a result, the experiential, feeling component of their work is diminished in importance. People become "a shoulder," or "a knee"; the breadth of their human experience is reduced to a number on a scale representing their level of pain.

Just as you need time to develop a relationship with your own body and let it communicate its sensations and the connectedness of its parts, your clients need your guidance to develop the ability to describe the emotions, sensations, and interconnections they feel in their own bodies. The ability to pay attention to and dialogue with internal sensations is something many people need to be taught. Body-therapy practitioners must ask themselves if they have this ability or even sense what it means. If they do not, they cannot encourage it in their clients.

Reading the Language of the Body

The language of the body is not verbal; the body speaks by means of sensation and changes in sensation. When you get on the ball, what you experience first is not your mind saying "I feel such and such," but a series of physical sensations. Only then does the mind pick up on the experience and seek a verbal expression of it.

Having a relationship with your body means being able to listen closely to different qualities of body messages—not simple "pain" or "pleasure," but different degrees of and changes in sensation. If you have some discomfort, can you feel a change in its intensity? Can you feel for connections between one body part and another? Can you look at your body and read the messages it is communicating—for example, can you recognize an alignment problem and the various ways it affects functioning? Can you feel when your body is sending signals of illness? This may sound simple; however, most people have no concept that it is possible to read body messages and recognize when something is wrong with their own bodies, even though the body has been sending signals all along. It is usually not until after the fact that most people begin to understand that the years-old contraction in their leg meant they might develop sciatica later on.

The classic example of this lack of awareness is when you hear: "He was the healthiest guy in the world, and he just suddenly dropped dead of a heart attack!" I know that before the heart attack this man had to have experienced pressure and pain in his chest; he likely experienced other symptoms as well, but he never paid attention to any of them. Most people in our society lack the education that would have enabled such a man to sort out his body messages and possibly prevent his heart attack. People need to be taught that subtle messages from the body are valid and important pieces of information.

The possibility of developing an astute awareness of body sensations is a central message of this book. Only when you are able to tell that something is wrong in your body can you take action to create a positive change.

Practitioners of Hanna Somatics, Feldenkrais, Body-Mind Centering, and other somatic therapies, who are dedicated to helping people acquire a deep inner awareness of their bodies, will already have developed the kind of relationship I have described. Similarly, because most forms of hatha yoga emphasize feeling the body releasing into postures as you hold them, people with a solid yoga background are likely to be able to sense inner change in their bodies. And since yoga affects so many parts of the body, yoga practitioners can also feel where and how their restrictions in a pose affect other parts of the body. (This is unlike other forms of exercise, in which the movements performed do not reveal restrictions unless a restriction is causing pain or reducing performance.) For practitioners who already have this kinesthetic awareness, Body Rolling is a tool for sharpening it and learning to utilize it directly in practice with clients. Body Rolling is a wonderful tool that all kinds of body-therapy practitioners can integrate into their current work. When a person has the ball at a certain part of the body and feels sensations in other parts, and then feels everything starting to release, his mind becomes captivated and begins trying to understand the experience.

For example, working with the ball may cause a release of tension that was unconsciously being held in a certain area. The body responds with a sudden letting go that is immediately registered by the brain as, "I didn't know I was holding so much there. What a relief!" Whereas your clients may work with Body Rolling to experience a general release that would reinforce the work you do in sessions together, body-therapy practitioners can get as detailed as they would like in developing this dialogue in sensation through Body Rolling, down to literally working each individual muscle from origin to insertion, feeling its quality, and sensing which muscles connect with it. To be a truly effective body-therapy practitioner and educator you need to develop this ability to feel the way muscle tissue releases in your own body.

As a rule, practitioners feel the quality of a muscle before they start working; then they work it; then they feel for a change in it. Many are unaware that it is also possible to feel a muscle releasing under the practitioner's fingers at the moment the release is occurring. A muscle worked at its origins knows the natural direction of release; there is actually a physical sensation as the muscle releases toward its insertion. At first the sensation is quite subtle, rather like the sigh within a deep breath. The muscle softens, and as the fibers begin to elongate toward their insertion you can sense the release of a pent-up energy that has been held at the origin and now streams through the muscle. Practitioners need to experience this letting-go process—both the sensation as it happens and the way the muscle feels afterward. It is this sensation of release that you want to transmit to clients.

Some practitioners might not be able at first to feel these subtle sensations. Often people are unsure of what they are feeling and fear they are making things up. With time, however, everybody can develop this strong kinesthetic sense of release. Body Rolling provides a solid, detailed, organized method for doing so, with the ball becoming a tool for self-study of your own anatomy. The more you do this type of exploration, the sooner you will see the effects in your practice. For example, say I am lying with the ball pressing into the adductors of my left leg. Suddenly I feel the external obliques releasing, and then my entire torso on that side releases and elongates. This tells me that shortness and tension in the adductors could cause contraction of the abdominal muscles, affecting origins and insertions from the pubic area up into my ribs. This in turn could shorten my torso and restrict movement. Having made this connection in my own body, when I work on someone with a contracted torso I will know to check this relationship between adductors and external obliques as one possible key to the solution of my client's problem.

To take a more complex example, suppose I am working the ball up from my sacrum into my lower back, and without moving any further up my back I begin to feel my shoulder releasing. The ball is not even at my shoulder. My brain, registering these changes, makes a connection between the lower back and the shoulder. If I did not know anatomy I would simply recognize that there was some kind of connection between my lower back and my shoulder. However, with my knowledge of anatomy I am aware that the latissimus dorsi begins in my lower back and inserts in my arm. This means that working to elongate the latissimus dorsi will begin to release the whole length of my back—that is, the quadratus lumborum, serratus posterior inferior, and trapezius muscles will also release. This series of releases demonstrates the principle that when you apply pressure to a muscle in the direction of its natural movement, all the muscles that have any connection to it will also begin to release. This pattern of releases is a manifestation of the body's innate intelligence.

Working in a Problem-Solving Mode

When you have a problem in your life, you use your mind to reason out a solution. You can address your body in the same way, and once you have learned how to use the ball as a tool for solving your own body's problems, you can use it to get others to really understand what is going on in their bodies as well.

Suppose a client comes in complaining of shortness of breath and a general sense of collapse on her left side. I invite her to roll up the right side; she objects that the problem is not on that side, and I suggest that there might be some connections. As she rolls up her right side, she is astonished to discover that she feels tremendous tightness there. She experiences a difference in muscle quality between the two sides that she never knew existed. We talk about the connection between the two sides. With this experience she can now see that, instead of just fixing the area where she feels the discomfort, the solution might involve balancing both sides of the body.

In Body Rolling we strive to create balance. For whatever reasons in life, people often rely on one side of the body to do most of their work. The muscles become much tighter on this side, which is often called our "strong" side. The stronger that side is, however, the more difficult it becomes for the other side to do its share of the work, so that other side becomes weaker. Once you start to release the working side, the weaker side can begin to take more responsibility.

This difference in quality between the two sides often signals the existence of discomfort. My client was aware of a problem on her left side *because* the tissues on her whole right side were hard as rock. Once we released the right side, the left side could function better. My client did not need to know the names of muscles to participate in this discovery; it was a whole-body pattern discovered simply through attending to sensation. Such discoveries are part of the experiential aspect of the ball work, and are gratifying for practitioner and client alike.

In Body Rolling it is essential to always treat both sides of the body in order to give the client the experiential education about what hurts and why. This is how the client becomes aware of the nature of her own posture and movements, what her body sensations are, and how these contribute to her well-being or lack of it. She can begin to question her common postural patterns and bring greater mindfulness to her patterns of sleeping, standing, sitting, working, or even talking on the phone. When I am working on someone's shoulder, he might tell me that he feels the effects of the work in his knee. His mind has made that connection. I can validate the reality of his perception by helping him see the possible relationships between shoulder and knee via his postural holding patterns, weight distribution, and ways of using his body in work or sports.

As you work more on yourself, feeling and exploring the different areas that might be key to a physical problem of your own and achieving good results, your insights grow sharper. This translates into more acute problem-solving in your practice. If you have investigated your own lower back discomfort, for example, when someone then comes to you with a lower back problem you will know which muscles above and below the lower back might need to be given length in order to relieve the discomfort. Following your hands-on assessment you can explain which muscles are involved in that person's pattern, how each of these muscles or muscle groups release, and how the person can work the area on his own to continue reaping the benefits of your session.

Working with Pain

Pain is a specific type of message that the body sends, one that you, and therefore your clients, can learn to work with. Rolling on the ball gives you the option to observe how you respond to pain. Pain may press your panic button and make you contract with the fear of experiencing more pain. But it is also possible when the ball hits a painful spot to say to yourself, "OK, this hurts. Let me stay here with it and breathe. Maybe it will dissolve." The pain might also provoke curiosity to explore it and find its source. By bringing your attention to the focal point of the pain and then using the breath as a focusing tool, you can feel the sensations of pain begin to shift, and oftentimes to subside.

People who have experienced intense or chronic pain often become so afraid of feeling it again that even a small degree of pain makes them panic and contract, which can bring on more pain. If you can ask that person, "Is it really that bad? If you stay there and breathe, does it get better or worse? Can you move around with the ball—does that change things?" she may discover that pain can change in quality and location. When a person has experienced a severe blow, after the initial healing takes place a protective layer sometimes builds up around the traumatized tissues, and that part of the body loses its feeling. The goal then becomes retrieving conscious awareness of sensation.

Another type of pain message is what some people consider a "good hurt." Although they feel discomfort, they sense that something positive is happening. This kind of sensation generally means that the body wants the ball to stay at the painful point and work through the pain. The body is saying, "Yes, go for it!" Soon where the client felt pain he now feels ease and a sense of space.

For people who were beaten or raped or have experienced any other such physical and emotional trauma, Body Rolling may be preferable to hands-on work. As therapists we are in a position of authority, to the degree that we or our clients choose to put us there. We are in the position of doing something *to* or *on* our clients—or at least our clients may perceive the relationship that way. With Body Rolling our clients can feel that they are doing the work themselves. They control how deeply they want to work, avoiding the areas of the body they do not feel ready to work on, or—if they are ready—confronting the feelings locked within these areas at their own pace.

Sometimes people do not tell you that they have experienced physical or sexual abuse, but there are common clues that an observant practitioner can pick up on. If I go to work on someone's pelvic area and see her contract through the pelvis and rotate her legs inward, or roll her eyes up into her head (a sign that she is losing contact with her body), I stop. I explain that this is an area of great contraction, and that whatever the reason her body has developed this strong holding pattern, it is essential to open up that area in order to relieve her pain. I explain further that she herself needs to understand why and how her body has gone into this contraction, which is what has caused the pain that brought her to me. As an educator, my role is to help her realize that she needs to go through the process of understanding how she has somatized an experience and learning what her body needs to transform that experience at the level of the tissues, and that if she does not take the responsibility to work on this problem herself, she will not be able to resolve it.

Then I suggest that, instead of having me work on her, she try working with the ball. I have her lie with the ball on the pubic bone and breathe, then let the ball roll just above the bone and see if she can let it sink into the belly. Then I ask her to roll on the ball toward the hip to one side, and then to the other side. I say, "Stay there and breathe. See how much release you can go for."

When someone openly tells me that she has been sexually or physically abused, I respond, "I can work on you, but then I'm another person *doing* something to you. It is very important that you yourself be the one to go into this area, confront your feelings, and be responsible for letting go of the trauma. This way you're not again placing yourself in a vulnerable position by letting someone else into an area that has already been traumatized." At the same time that I encourage this level of self-work, it is important that I stay very present and support my client in her process.

How to Use the Breath

When you watch a baby you can see its entire body expanding and contracting from pelvis to head as it breathes. Soon, however, usually by the time the child begins walking, that elasticity is lost and breathing becomes compartmentalized. The breathing pattern roots deeper and deeper, so that by the time they are adults most people breathe only from the chest; some take only minute breaths just from the upper chest. These people may never know what it is to take a deep breath. On the other end of the spectrum, those who have had some yoga training usually just breathe abdominally. (One group likely to breathe more fully are those who have had voice training.) The more breathing is inhibited, the less people can understand the importance of the breath to their well-being. They are aware that, physiologically speaking, we cannot live without breathing, but beyond that they have no idea of the function of the breath.

People who teach others how to breathe may talk about breathing for relaxation but they do not always stress its importance as a tool for correcting and improving structure. In fact, the breath can be used internally as a powerful tool for releasing individual muscles.

What the ball does is give people a real experience of how critical breathing is for increasing well-being. You can restore to the body the elasticity of infancy and expand the entire area from your head to the tip of the coccyx with the breath—in fact, you can guide the breath into your left shoulder, or your right hip, or anywhere else in the body.

Since most people never consciously think about breathing, telling them how they should breathe instantly produces feelings of inadequacy, because they likely do not understand what you mean. The ball provides a point to breathe into; it is a powerful tool for body-mind focus because you can feel it. As we settle into working a particular area, I say to my clients, "See if you can inhale and visualize pushing your body out against the ball with the breath. Then as you exhale let the weight of your body sink into the ball." As they do this, they begin to see that they can direct their breath to specific parts of the body. They feel the effect of inhaling and exhaling, and they feel the results: tight, tense muscle softens. Thus they learn experientially that the breath can be a major healing tool.

Some clients who are locked into old breathing patterns find it very difficult to breathe into specific areas of the body. To them I say, "Send the breath to the point where the ball is. If you cannot get it there, *visualize* that you're getting it there.

Eventually you will get it there." When the ball reaches an area where they can breathe more freely, they feel the greater muscle release in that area. This difference enables them to understand the importance of breathing.

The breath is an extremely valuable tool for releasing tension because pushing the breath out into the ball creates expansion and release from the inside out, addressing the fact that people can be tight on the outside but have no strength inside. Working from the inside out focuses attention on expanding the lungs. As people attempt to do this they feel the inner muscles that allow for outward expansion. This motion begins to release those deeply held internal muscles.

Aberrations in breathing patterns are often a result of issues of self-image, as well as a child's mirroring of her parents, for breathing patterns are closely connected to emotions and psychological imprinting. For example, children who are physically beaten or shouted at develop a tight rib cage. The rib cage is our natural armor, protecting the heart and lungs; the more armor there is in the thoracic area, the more breathing is inhibited. Although the rib cage is our protective shield, it does not have to restrict our movement through life. Once we realize that our protective shield no longer serves us, and that an open, flexible rib cage will serve us better, it becomes possible to let go of that armoring and work to free the rib cage. Ultimately, greater lung expansion, greater flexibility of the thoracic cage, and the resulting greater movement of the head, neck, shoulders, and arms make possible more complete expression of our true being.

A common effect of self-image on breathing patterns in our culture is that women in particular walk around trying to look thin. Many women who are heavy on the bottom contract the upper half of their bodies in an attempt to feel smaller. One client of mine had had her weight under control for a while but then started gaining weight again. Looking in the mirror, she felt angry with herself. The more angry and frustrated she became, the more she tried to make herself small by contracting all her intercostal muscles and her diaphragm. Someone who does that for twenty years and never breathes into her chest experiences minimum expansion in her lungs. As a result, her body cannot move. Pain patterns begin to develop.

A contracted rib cage in men is likely to be the result of the typical Napoleon posture. The shoulders are squared off and the back of the thoracic cage narrows and contracts inward, becoming immobile. This forces the rib cage to expand in front, but the intercostal muscles remain contracted and rigid. Such a man needs to learn how to expand the lungs so that the rib cage can soften and relax downward, freeing the neck and shoulders.

Most people only use one-quarter of their lung capacity. But if the lungs are not expanded to at least 50 percent of their capacity, there will be restriction throughout the torso. Considering how much anatomical space the lungs actually take up, you can see how great a possibility of expansion the chest area actually has. The entire thoracic area should expand on inhalation and relax on exhalation, like an accordion moving in and out. The more the lungs expand, the more open the whole thorax becomes and the more stimulation the muscles receive, since they are all stretching and contracting during respiration. In fact, you can use the breath to elongate all the muscles of the entire torso, including the individual abdominal muscles and the muscles of the back. In doing so you also stimulate organ function.

Remembering our goal of giving all muscles their maximum length, it is clear why working with the breath is essential in all the Body Rolling routines. For it is impossible to fully elongate the muscles of the torso if you are not consciously involving your respiration—just try raising your arms with your rib cage immobilized or "frozen." Many people who suffer from chronic neck and shoulder problems do not understand that these problems are related to lack of mobility in the torso—you cannot get full length through the neck if your thoracic cage is restricted. Unrestricted full-body breathing is also a key for eliminating tension and pressure in the head that may cause headaches.

Body Rolling teaches what yogis have understood for centuries: The breath is the most important tool for directing vital energy. Try doing the Body Rolling routines described in parts 2 and 3 first without breathing, and then focusing on full-body breathing. You will feel the power of the breath in helping move the body toward a profound experience of change.

CHAPTER

3

MAKING THE
MIND-BODY
CONNECTION

The connection between mind and body can be experienced in various modes: through the intellect, the emotions, or the vital energy.

Experiencing the Mind-Body
Through the Intellect

One goal of my body-therapy practice is to help people realize that they can use the intellect to understand what is going on in the body. For most people, the intellect is focused outside the body; they use the intellect only to deal with external events, such as problems at work. Using the rational mind to problem-solve with the body in the manner described in chapter 2 is completely foreign to them. However, it is a valuable skill, one I feel needs to be developed.

We all learn problem-solving skills as children, but only in restricted applications. Consequently, when physical problems arise, most people panic and run straight to doctors or body-therapy practitioners, those considered to be the body-problem solvers.

To me, this response is amazingly unnatural. The fact that people do not automatically and intuitively investigate their own bodies first to explore what might be wrong tells me that something inside them has become disconnected.

Certainly when I push clients by asking a lot of questions, they can eventually come up with a description of what they think is going on in their bodies. And, no matter how elementary their descriptions of the problem may be, they will be right. Yet, because they have never before applied their problem-solving abilities to the body process, they grow embarrassed as they try to describe their sensations. They are awkward and uncertain, like very young children being questioned in school.

Still more confounding to me is the fact that this type of problem-solving is also foreign to some body-therapy practitioners. Frequently, body-therapy practitioners are trained to simply perform a technique rather than to look at the whole person in an analytical way. Consequently, many body-therapy practitioners are in the same situation as my clients, having themselves never applied their problem-solving abilities to their bodies.

It is extremely important to listen to the way people describe the entirety of their experience of discomfort, including the other parts of the body that they feel to be affected. Their descriptions enhance what you learn from observing and from touching them, giving you an enormous amount of information to begin your problem-solving process. What a client says about her complaint is important, because it is *her* body at issue. Having her description of discomfort acknowledged also teaches her that she does get messages from the body that she can sort out herself, without specialized knowledge. For these reasons I tell my clients that if a practitioner they go to does not want first-person input on what the client thinks is going on in the body, *they should walk out.*

LEVELS OF INTERACTION

The intellect interacts with the body at several levels. On one level, the mind is completely detached from the information the body is giving. Many forms of exercise encourage this lack of connection. Because fitness is fashionable and people know intellectually that cardiovascular exercise is important, they feel obliged to partake in some form of exercise, so they dutifully run, cycle, or use a treadmill. But if you look into the bicycle room in most gyms, you see about one-third of the exercisers reading or watching television as they "ride." Similarly, many runners listen to music or motivational tapes while they clock their miles. All this fitness activity—performed in a spirit of getting it over with—simply perpetuates the body-mind split that characterizes most of our daily activities. And it is when people perform physical exercise with their minds separate from their motions that most fitness injuries occur.

At the second level of body-mind connection, the mind receives some kinesthetic information about what is happening in the body, and therefore the mind becomes more present in the activity. When the instructor in an aerobics class tells you that a particular stretch works the hamstrings, your brain takes note of it, and you think, "Okay, I'm working my hamstrings!" But the recognition is still separate from the action. When you bend over and do the stretch, your body's message is, "This hurts," but you do not know why it hurts.

If the mind has more information, however, instead of just registering discomfort it can observe the whole muscle. When you put a ball under your sitzbone, where all the hamstring muscles originate, and roll through those muscles down the leg, toward their insertion points on the tibia and fibula, you are experiencing the hamstrings release along their entire length. Now the message is, "I can feel the muscle elongating."

In order to create this type of connection in which body and mind dialogue with one another, the physical sensation must be translated into words *and* the body must fully experience what the mind is being told. For example, I might tell a client that he is experiencing pain because his hip is rotated and the muscles are tight on one side and loose on the other side. While his mind can understand that description intellectually, it is not until I touch him and he actually has the body experience I am describing verbally that he will make the body-mind connection.

Once the mind can register and describe the body sensations that result from rolling on the ball, it can reason about these results. As my client rolls through the different muscle groups of the leg, he can feel which of those muscles are tighter because he experiences that tightness as greater discomfort. But he can also deduce that these must be the muscles holding his hip in that rotated position and that releasing them might relieve the pain in his hip. This is the third level of connection.

You can help people develop the body-mind connection by suggesting all the different possible interrelationships between body systems and parts while you work on them. The more you do this, the more familiarity the client has with making the body-mind connection. Soon the connected body-mind is second nature to him. And Body Rolling gives the client a tool to expand this awareness on his own.

A final component of helping clients develop the body-mind connection is empowering them to understand all the aspects of their lives that might contribute to their physical problems. You begin to question people about their work, sports, or hobbies to see how these activities might be affecting them. Then you help them really understand what muscles and postural changes are involved, to the point where they acquire a fairly complete understanding of how their complaint developed and how it needs to be worked on. Ultimately you encourage them to take this capacity for reasoning about the body and use it in all types of physical experience.

RELAXATION AND THE INTELLECT

Most people are generally aware that, in order to function well and stay healthy in our stressful society, they should learn to relax. But I find that, for many people, relaxation is only an intellectual concept. Simply lying down and closing your eyes does not equal relaxing. Relaxation occurs when the mind is drawn into a letting-go process that the body undergoes; the more fully the body releases, the more completely the mind becomes involved. This is how the stilling of the mind occurs.

To understand the relaxation response, people need something they can feel. In Body Rolling, the ball becomes the bridge between body and mind. The sensation of breathing into the point where the ball is resting gives the mind the physical focus that allows it to become absorbed in the body's messages of relaxation: muscles and joints releasing, the slowing of the breath, and so on. Even people with no experience of bodywork or relaxation exercises stop being impatient and restless when they get down on the ball, for they make this mind-body connection and are drawn into deep states of relaxation.

Experiencing the Mind-Body Through the Emotions

A second mode of mind-body connection occurs by way of the emotions, which arise through body experience. Often touching a client at a particular point on the body evokes a sensation that sparks an emotion and the memory of a past experience. The mind is drawn to engage in this somatic experience, recalling the exact experience or experiences that became lodged at that point and interpreting them.

Body-therapy practitioners know that everyone has contracted places in their bodies where they hold specific emotions—areas that tickle or where they cannot stand to be touched, or tissues that are immediately affected by an upsetting situation. When these places are touched, emotions arise. Many people feel that they cannot let someone else touch these areas of the body, but they can touch themselves there. If they can stay there, focusing the breath, their own healing energy allows the blocked emotions to release.

Work on the abdomen, for example, often releases the diaphragm. The release registers as a sharp pain that may quickly bring up sadness or some other emotion. As you work on the ball, you can stay there and let the emotion come out, or you can choose to not deal with it at that moment and roll to the next point. If you do let yourself experience this emotion, the body begins to breathe more deeply. The area being pressed by the ball softens, and so does the pain; then the emotion, too, softens and releases.

Body-therapy practitioners will often identify a spot on a client where an emotional block is tightening the tissues, and press directly into it. This is likely to bring up a sudden outburst of tears or other expression of emotion. The release may be a good thing, but it occurs in a shocking, explosive way as panic enters that body area and the emotion bursts out. The client feels caught off guard. To achieve the same result in a less alarming way, when you begin to sense that emotions are blocking an area of the body, think in terms of creating space there, as you can do with the ball, instead of exerting pressure on the spot. The space allows the blocked emotions room to move around and loosen up. They can then emerge in a more peaceful way, and in their own time.

Experiencing in your own body the way in which creating space can soften emotional release will suggest ways to facilitate this experience for your clients. Sometimes, for example, you will be working on someone and find you cannot get through certain muscles. Those tissues will not release because you are working on them only on a physical level. But if you give your client a ball and encourage her to roll through those tissues herself, she can stay at that area, breathing, and feeling whatever is being held soften and release its grip.

Once people have experienced the connection between tight places in the body and held-in emotions, they can interpret the body's signals to become more aware of their feelings. They realize that the body is more than a mechanism that moves you around; it is a powerful tool for developing increased self-awareness.

Experiencing the Mind-Body Through the Vital Energy

According to yogic philosophy, our reservoir of vital energy is located at the base of the spine, in the perineal area. The ultimate goal of hatha yoga is to remove all the blockages that prevent this energy from flowing freely up and down the spine. When you roll the ball slowly from the coccyx over the sacrum, as in the basic back routine (see chapter 5), you are opening channels for that healing energy to move up the spine and, via the nerve roots, out into the rest of the body.

The spine is the major pathway along which we can direct our vital energy through the body. As you roll up the spine, you can visualize at each point that you are opening that area, elongating all the muscles and creating space between the vertebrae so that energy can flow as freely as possible. It is important to understand that each of us has this life force—chi, vital energy, or kundalini—which, when tapped into, can be a powerful tool for self-healing and self-awareness.

In this mode of connection through energy, your mind remains very present as you roll, and as your energy moves up the spine it acts almost as a guide, releasing your muscles and making a pathway for the ball. You experience a flooding sensation that moves up the spine, along with a sense of deep release and relaxation that fills your whole being with healing energy.

The beauty of this experience is that it makes you aware that your own energy, guided by the routine, is doing your own healing. And it is a revelation to realize that, if you have so much healing energy inside you, so do your clients. Which means that you do not have to work so hard—in fact, your work will only go so far in moving another toward well-being. You must tap into your client's own energy in order for true healing to occur.

Waking up this energy may take some time. We spend much of our daily lives sitting right on the spot where this energy reservoir is located. Whenever there has been a lot of weight bearing down upon the region between the ischium and the coccyx or sacrum, you may need to roll from the tip of the coccyx up one side of the sacrum three or four times before the sacrum is ready to allow the energy to move up and release to happen. (Chapter 5 will cover this routine in detail.) It is important to focus on the intention of moving up the sacrum slowly point by point, not skipping any spaces. If you roll too fast you might skip over a blocked area, and the flow of energy would be obstructed there.

Once you have this energy experience, you may start to wonder: Am I giving this to my clients? And if not, do I need to change the way I work? Can I teach this to my clients so they can encourage their own self-healing? Such questions may bring up a challenge: When you become aware of how much people can do to promote their own healing, you realize that your clients might not need to work with you as often. If you truly want to empower people, your role, as well as being a body practitioner, might be to become this kind of an educator or facilitator.

Working Toward the "Deep Sink"

Initially, Body Rolling is like an exercise class; starting at the grossest physical level, you simply follow the prescribed movements, which affect the most superficial muscles. As these muscles release, you begin to address deeper muscle layers. When these deeper tissues free up, you affect still deeper ones. Take the layers of the erector spinae muscles, for example. Each time you do the back routine you are working more deeply, with more focus and intention, and affecting a deeper muscle layer. The freer these layers of tissue become, the closer you get to the level of pure energy.

Body Rolling requires persistent effort as you move from layer to layer; ultimately, it can take you to a very profound level of experience. After you have worked with the ball for a while and have released the more superficial muscle-holding patterns, the rhythm of the release process speeds up. The body takes over and moves the releasing along on its own. It is as though the body becomes conditioned to the ball; as soon as the ball touches you, your breathing deepens and the muscles begin to release and stretch without the mind needing to direct the process at all.

Once you have eliminated all the blockages along the spine and your energy is flowing freely, the ball work enters the profound stage I call the "deep sink." The mind clicks off, and you move beyond sense messages such as pain and pleasure into a realm of pure body sensation—a state of great peace and profound relaxation beyond body and mind. This is the highest level of the mind-body connection, the level at which the two become one. It is the same state people try to achieve through stress-reduction techniques, such as meditation, visualization, and biofeedback. Often they fail because of the difficulty of mental concentration. But with Body Rolling, the body takes you there.

Now that you understand the philosophy and basic principles of Body Logic and Body Rolling, you can go on to part 2 to begin exploring the basics of Body Rolling. Once you become familiar with the basic routines described in chapters 5 through 7, you can consult the chapters in part 3 to work with specific conditions and in greater depth.

I urge you to use this book as a tool for your own growth and self-exploration. There is a saying that you can only take someone as far along a path as you have traveled yourself. The more self-work you do with Body Rolling, the better able you will be to guide your clients toward full body/self awareness.

PART TWO

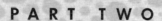

$\mathcal{T}$HE BASICS

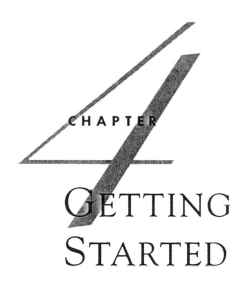

CHAPTER

GETTING
STARTED

Part 2 gets you started with Body Rolling. This chapter covers guidelines for beginning your own explorations and for teaching Body Rolling to your clients. The next three chapters present basic routines to lengthen the torso. Giving length to the torso eliminates 90 percent of the discomforts clients present to you. You will also be using these routines and variations on them to treat specific conditions.

Choosing the Right Ball

Body Rolling is practiced on a hollow ball. People who are 5'1" and shorter need a six- to nine-inch-diameter ball; those who are taller should use a nine- to ten-inch ball. Six-inch balls are also useful for more detailed work in such areas as the neck and armpit.

When I first began teaching Body Rolling I thought almost any type of ball would work, but experience taught me otherwise. Different balls have different qualities.

People may use the cheap vinyl balls found in drugstores, but these lack adequate density and resistance, and they cannot be reinflated. Inflatable utility balls, available at sporting goods and toy stores, usually are more durable. They have better density, but little resistance. However, you will not get optimal results with either of these balls, and anyone weighing over 180 pounds cannot use them because the ball will bend out of shape and not provide any benefit at all.

Based on the feedback I received from clients I designed a set of reinflatable balls that have the right densities, resistances, and weight-bearing capacities for different bodies, including softer balls for people who have injuries or bone problems. The more you sink into one of these balls, the more deeply it will press into the area of the body that you are focusing on. Such a ball lets you separate each individual vertebra from its neighbors; you can also isolate specific muscles. These balls are also better for working on bone; they can penetrate intervertebral spaces and exert a level of pressure that changes the quality of bone. See the resource section at the back of the book for mail order information.

Eight to ten inches is the best size for working on the spine. For work on the abdomen and shoulders, six- to nine-inch balls are better. When rolling up the side, for instance, you might start with a nine-inch ball and then switch to a smaller ball when you reach the armpit. The smaller ball will fit more closely into that space. **Never use *any* six-inch ball on the side between the hips and ribs; it can break your floating ribs.**

People who are frail, lack flexibility, are not physically active, or those who have structural problems or little muscle mass, should start their practice of Body Rolling with a softer, nine- to ten-inch ball. **Drugstore balls, and any other hard balls, are not safe for anyone with any bone abnormality, such as osteoporosis or another form of spinal rigidity.** As a general rule, when someone finds a ball painful to roll over, that ball is too hard for the person.

Never let anyone use a volleyball, basketball, golf ball, or weighted (medicine) ball for Body Rolling. Doing so would be exteremely dangerous and could cause serious injury.

Heavy people can practice Body Rolling with a ball that is strong enough to take their weight. The balls I've designed can hold up to 350 pounds, and I have gotten three-hundred-pound people to work successfully with the ball.

In general, you should not let clients with structural problems begin working with the ball before you have described to them what they need from it, given them detailed instructions for working with it, and determined which ball is safe for them to start with. You will also need to create the mood and set the pace, showing them how to work slowly and use the breath and the weight of the body to create space. It is impossible to do all this in the last five minutes of a bodywork session. Therefore, I usually schedule one session with my clients specifically for the ball work, so I can ensure that they really understand it.

What to Wear

The ball slips less on skin than on clothing, but for some people the sensation of the ball directly on the skin is irritating. Since loose clothing will get in the way as you roll, the best attire is a leotard with or without tights. Tee shirts, even when tucked in, tend to bunch up behind the ball as it rolls. People with long hair should tie it up to prevent it from getting caught under the ball.

Body Rolling is best done with some kind of padding on the floor, such as an exercise mat or carpet. A yoga sticky mat is particularly good for keeping the ball from slipping out from under you.

How Much Time Does It Take?

For body-therapy practitioners, Body Rolling has two applications. It is a self-help tool, a workout you can do at the end of the day to unwind and release your work patterns from your body; it takes twenty to thirty minutes to roll up both sides and the center of your spine. Body Rolling is also a form of self-exploration. For this purpose, you need to set aside a larger block of time in order to explore your muscular holding patterns in detail.

For your clients, a typical routine—such as rolling up each side of the back and up the center of the spine, or rolling up each side of the body and up the center of the back—should take between twenty-five and thirty-five minutes. Some clients will claim that they only have fifteen minutes to spend on a Body Rolling routine. Even in this short period of time they can simply roll up the center of the spine and still receive benefits. Clients working to relieve the various conditions described in part 3 will need to devote more time to each session, but they can limit their practice to three times a week.

As you continue Body Rolling, however, the time factor changes. The more you do it, the more quickly you can connect to the energy in your spine, and the shorter your sessions become. This is because when there is more congestion in the body, the energy travels more slowly. The more toned and released muscles are, the quicker they respond. In the beginning you might need to stay longer at each point to really feel a change occur. But once your body gets used to doing Body Rolling and you work through the more superficial muscle layers, release happens much faster.

A Basic Rule

Body Rolling is extremely powerful work, and one rule is critical: If you roll up one side of the body you must always work the other side as well, even if you are doing the routine because just one side is hurting. This rule applies to the legs as well as to the torso. For this reason, you should always end a session by working up the spine. Increased length achieved in other areas of the body must be matched in the spine in order to keep the body balanced. For example, sometimes one side of the body will release more than the other. Working up the center of the spine at the end of the session will create releases on both sides, balancing them according to my theory that as you bear your body weight onto a bone via the ball, you release every muscle that has an attachment to that bone.

Rolling up the spine at the end of a session also allows a much deeper overall release. Working up the sides, for example, elongates all the muscles that give length to the torso. Although the spine also gets some additional length from these muscles, on the final roll the deeper erector spinae muscles can let go even further, creating still greater intervertebral space in the torso.

Working both sides has an additional advantage. People cannot experience change unless they have some basis for comparison. In Body Rolling you roll up one side, then compare it to the side you have not done. Lying on the floor after working the first side, you may notice that you are breathing differently. The way your body rests on the floor or the way you walk and stand after you get up may also have changed. This comparison teaches people to distinguish subtle sensations that signal changes in the quality of their tissues.

Getting Comfortable on the Ball

As in any new form of exercise or movement, it takes a while to get comfortable with Body Rolling, so here are several pointers to keep in mind in the early stages.

First, it helps to remember that there is no single correct position for any of the routines. What is most important is that you feel balanced and comfortable on the ball. When first using the ball, people are often afraid that they will slide off. If the suggested position for a given routine does not make a person feel supported, I encourage finding another position that is comfortable. The main concern is to maintain awareness of letting the body weight sink into the ball, so that you are not holding yourself up in tension at the point where the ball is.

Sometimes, to get adequate pressure on the ball, as in working the legs or the sides of the body, you will need to lift your body weight with your arms and hold it for a while. This extra effort could cause a buildup of tension in the arms and shoulders. However, since you should always end a session by rolling up the back, you will ultimately release any tension in the neck or shoulders.

Another thing to keep in mind is that in certain parts of the body, such as the front of the thigh, the muscles tend to be attached to the bone and to each other. As you sink into the ball, you can expect to experience discomfort as the individual muscles begin to separate from each other and from the bone. This may feel as though the muscles are tensing up, but it is actually a reaction to the weight of the body on the ball affecting an already existing pattern of tension. Stay with it and you will feel the muscles release and free themselves.

Presenting Body Rolling to Clients

Every client will benefit greatly from any of the basic Body Rolling routines, which help maintain releases achieved in bodywork sessions. Before deciding exactly how to present Body Rolling, however, you need to size your client up, finding out what kind of person he is and how much time his schedule can realistically allow for routines.

If someone insists that he has no time and you can feel tension and contraction in his tissue, giving him a routine he cannot do will only make him feel guilty. You can encourage this highly stressed man just to roll up the center of his spine, taking ten to fifteen minutes to do so. Suggest that he do this routine, accompanied by soothing music, just before going to bed. (This practice is wonderful to recommend to anyone who has trouble getting to sleep.)

To enable clients to do Body Rolling effectively, you must educate them not only about how to do it but also about why they should do it. It is absolutely essential to stress the importance of their involvement in their own healing process, and to point out that work at home will facilitate the work being done with you.

If you tell people to do an exercise without explaining and demonstrating it sufficiently, most clients will just go through the motions and not get any benefits. But if you tell them that they bear the ultimate responsibility for their own healing and explain why working with the ball is an essential aspect of this self-work, you will instill in them the desire to do the routines, and this understanding will stay in their minds as they work.

Once clients have the motivation, they will want as much detailed information as they can absorb. This does not mean you must give muscle-specific instructions. Often when you give people technical anatomical terms they become anxious, worrying about forgetting the names and doing something wrong. All you need is a formula such as, "In this area, this is what we're trying to achieve." Thus, for someone who has lower back pain, you do not need to explain where the quadratus lumborum is and how to work it. Instead, just say that you want to create as much length as possible between the pelvis and the ribs to take any compression out of the lower back.

One thing I have learned during my nearly twenty years in this field is that Murphy's Law applies in bodywork as in other areas of life: If clients can do something wrong, they will. So when you give clients a routine to do at home, start with the simplest version. Then at the next session, ask what happened. Did they have pain? Did they sense an improvement in their condition? What did they feel while doing the routines?

Based on their responses, you can discern their level of awareness and how comfortable they were with the routine. Then, if appropriate, you can give them a little more detail, such as an additional task within the basic routine. You might say: "Now that you are comfortable rolling up the center of the spine, let's see if you can begin to feel the ball separating one vertebra from the next. Instead of creating space between the hips and rib cage in a general way, we now want to create intervertebral space."

Using a skeleton model or a diagram of the lumbar spine, you then show clients what an individual vertebra looks like and how rolling from one to the next would be achieved. With this intention in mind, and using the image of the vertebrae to visualize what is happening, the next time your clients roll up the spine they can feel for the sensation of the individual vertebrae.

To provide further support, talk them through the routine during a session. As you explain how to move, breathe, and sink into each spot, you are also setting a mood and tone, creating a relaxation experience. As clients begin to feel relaxed and you describe the details you want them to focus on, you are also observing them and helping them through the routine with hands-on guidance, if necessary.

Learning new movement activities makes some people nervous; they find translating verbal instructions into body movements quite difficult. But if you are there answering questions and generally making the experience easier, they will feel more confident when they go home. For the same reason, it is useful to work both sides of the body during the session. While doing the first side, help your clients get comfortable with the routine, then let them try it on their own working the second side.

Your role as body therapist is also to reinforce the validity of clients' sensations. People usually do not know what they are supposed to feel in an exercise like Body Rolling. It is all very new to those who are not body-oriented; they have no idea what it feels like when a muscle releases or elongates. This is where you relay your own experiential work with the ball. From your own experience of doing the routines, you can describe to clients what physical sensations might likely be experienced when muscles begin to let go. Soon they will be able to feel different types of subtle sensations in their own bodies.

Order and Pacing

Part of your educational role is to make it clear to clients that muscle release occurs in a natural order. To help them understand the importance of beginning at the base of the spine, give them the image that the muscles of the back are like the branches of a tree and must be activated from the roots. As the energy awakens, the muscles release, and this release grows as the ball moves up the spine.

This explanation will help clients understand that the body's energy does not just suddenly awaken, and that rolling quickly around the spine will not create the type of release they are after. Emphasize that Body Rolling is not about racing up the spine; it is rather about taking time for themselves. They really must focus mentally at each point on the sacrum, then breathe and wait. Guiding them with your voice, you can demonstrate the best pacing, which is to wait with one full, deep breath at each point, focusing on sending the breath into the point where the ball is. Encourage them to sit at each point, really letting their weight sink into it, concentrating on a deep inhalation, and then giving a long exhalation while letting the tissue sink deeper into the ball. In this way clients will experience how much time is required to truly begin feeling relaxed.

The routines that follow, including those in part 3 for specific problems, are addressed to you, the practitioner. The basic routines in part 2 also include sections on giving that routine to clients, illustrating how you can give instructions that are detailed yet also nonspecific and easy for a client with no anatomical knowledge to understand. I address these chapters to you, the practitioner, with the expectation that you will try each one on your own body and understand it anatomically before giving it to your clients. It is absolutely essential that you know each routine from firsthand experience, whether you personally have the relevant problem or not. That way, when you give this routine to a client, you can be both clear and convincing. Say you are treating a client with sciatica. Your experience of the sciatica routine will inform your explanation to the client, and you will be able to convey it without needing to speak in technical terms. For example, you might explain touch-and-tell anatomy this way: "These are the areas the nerve passes through and where the possible muscle constriction is, and this is why we roll through the whole buttock and then down the muscles of the leg, giving space to the whole affected area, taking pressure off the nerve and allowing it to heal." Only when you know the routine through experiencing it in your own tissue can you teach it to others.

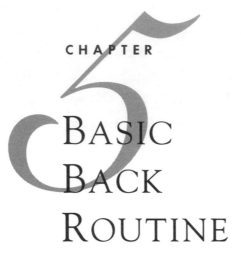

BASIC
BACK
ROUTINE

Bodywork therapies usually place great emphasis on working soft tissue. Since the key to a healthy body is a healthy spine, however, I emphasize working close to the spine. By doing so you can stimulate and tone the nervous system, thereby affecting more of the organism than if you work soft tissue alone.

In the basic back routines, you first roll up each side of the spine and then you roll up the center. As you roll up the sides of the spine you release the superficial muscles that begin at its base. Then, when you roll up the center, the deeper layer of erector spinae muscles that attach to the spinous and transverse processes release laterally in both directions.

Most of the time during exercise, and in life in general, people do not differentiate between the two sides of the back. Body Rolling gives them the opportunity to feel for differences in quality between the two sides, and between a specific area on one side and the same area on the other.

In general, people tend to use one side of the body more than the other. Right-handed people have more strength and muscle development on the right side, and left-handed people are more developed on the left side. When you take time to roll up each side of the spine, you really begin to experience how different the two sides are. As you begin investigating why this is so, you gradually grow more conscious about how you use each side. You begin to question the postures you hold while working, during exercise, and when relaxing at home. The ball enables you to sense for the first time the differences in quality between areas that are tight and other areas that can breathe, be flexible, and let go.

Recall the woman with discomfort on her left side, described in chapter 2, who discovered that it is actually much easier to roll up her left side than up her right side. At this point her mind kicks in: "Wow, the left side is where I hurt but the right side is more painful to go into! There must be an imbalance between the sides. Maybe my right side is tight to compensate for a weakness on the left. Or maybe my left side is painful because the right side is overworked and does not allow the left to work efficiently."

Feeling the differences side to side in this way sparks people's curiosity about what is going on in their bodies and why. This is the beginning of self-exploration and the realization that they can develop self-awareness and become responsible for the body's well-being. The concept that they can help themselves can then take root cellularly.

Rolling up one side can sometimes make the other side release quicker. Some areas that are holding on one side of the body may not release at all until you roll up the other side. Once you experience whatever release each side will give and then roll up the center, you will achieve a far deeper final release.

Self-Exploration for the Practitioner

UP THE TWO SIDES OF THE SPINE

Sit on the ball so that it presses on the point between the two sitzbones and the tip of the coccyx (figure 5.1). Roll downward on the right side, angling the ball into the ischium (figure 5.2). Roll around on the ischium a bit. This movement begins to loosen the origins of the adduc-

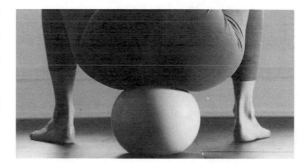

FIGURE 5.1

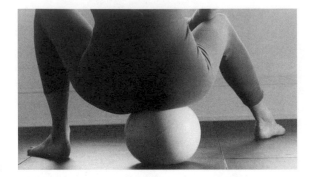

FIGURE 5.2

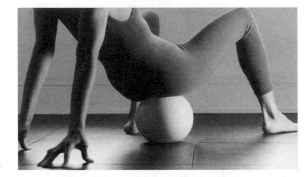

FIGURE 5.3

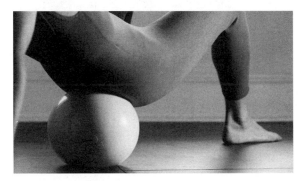

FIGURE 5.4

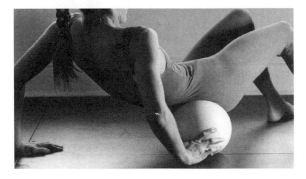

FIGURE 5.5

tor magnus and the hamstrings—the semimembranosus, semitendinosus, and biceps femoris muscles. From there, roll upward at an angle to the tip of the coccyx, so that the ball is exerting pressure on the right side of the coccyx (figure 5.3).

Now, with the weight of your body pressing into the ball, begin rolling it upward, tracing a continuous line up the sacrum over the right sacroiliac joint (figure 5.4), stopping every one-half to one inch. Make sure the ball is angling toward the sacrum, not the ilium. Breathe at each point: on the inhalation, bring breath down into the spot where the ball is; on the exhalation, let your weight sink into the ball.

Trace all the way up to the top of the sacrum. Moving along this line from the coccyx to the top of the sacrum, you will be initiating release of the gluteus maximus at its origin, and of the latissimus dorsi, which connects to the sacrum via the thoracolumbar fascia. Gently roll the ball outward along the iliac crest (figure 5.5). Keeping the ball at the most lateral point of the iliac crest, (figure 5.6; you might need to hold the ball with your hand in order to stay at this point), focus on spreading and separating the ilium away from the sacrum. Breathe into this point, which is the origin of the quadratus lumborum. Creating space here will allow you to insert the ball more easily between the sacrum and L5.

Now roll the ball horizontally toward the spine, crossing the muscle fibers of the quadratus lumborum. Applying pressure on this muscle creates length in the lower back.

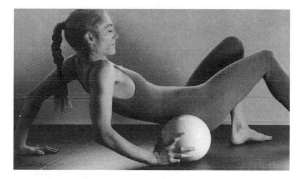

FIGURE 5.6

At the spine, place the ball between S1 and L5, tilting your body to the right to apply pressure on the right side of the spine (figure 5.7). Here you are creating space between the sacrum and the lumbar spine. As you move up from L5 to L4, you are stimulating release at the insertion points of the quadratus lumborum along

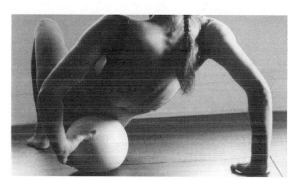

FIGURE 5.7

the transverse processes of the lumbar vertebrae. Each time you inhale, expand your breath and bring it to this area. As you exhale, sink into the ball so that it lifts up under L4, separating L4 from L5. Keep in mind the image of spreading the pelvis away from the sacrum, so that as you breathe you are widening your lower back.

When you feel that you have created this separation, roll the ball slightly upward, pushing it against L3. Continue rolling up the five lumbar vertebrae, releasing all the insertion points of the quadratus lumborum. As you focus on this deeper muscle, you are also initiating release of the lowermost origin points of the latissimus dorsi at the sacral and iliac crests and the thoracolumbar fascia. Giving length here to the latissimus dorsi, the longest muscle of the back, will stimulate the lengthening and upward release of the deeper back muscles: the serratus posterior inferior, the transverse abdominis, the trapezius, and the erector spinae. These releases in turn will stimulate a chain of releases all the way up the back.

At L3 you reach the serratus posterior inferior, which overlies the quadratus lumborum. After rolling up the five lumbar vertebrae on the right side, go back to L3. To release the serratus posterior inferior you must change the angle of the ball, directing

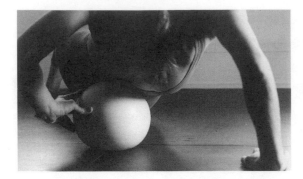

FIGURE 5.8

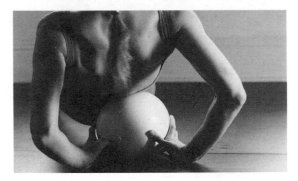

FIGURE 5.9

its pressure into the origin point of the muscle on L3 (figure 5.8) and then rolling outward from L3 to the muscle's insertion point at the inferior border of the twelfth rib (figure 5.9). Repeat this rolling up the length of the serratus posterior inferior from L2 to the eleventh rib, L1 to the tenth rib, and T11 and T12 to the ninth rib. Really breathe into this muscle, bringing breath into and spreading the lowest back ribs. Your image here is of spreading the ribs horizontally.

Contraction of the quadratus lumborum will pull the serratus posterior inferior and the rib cage downward toward the pelvis. A contracted serratus posterior inferior narrows the rib cage in toward the spine, restricting the movement of the breath into the back of the ribs. Contraction of both of these muscles initially causes extreme stiffness in the lower back. If the contraction becomes chronic, it can lead to serious lower back problems, such as a herniated disk.

Roll the ball back in toward the spine, to the origin of the trapezius at T12. Begin rolling the ball up the thoracic spine one vertebra at a time, trying to keep the ball pressing into the space between the spinous process and the transverse process on the right side of the spine, then angling it upward and outward to follow the direction of the

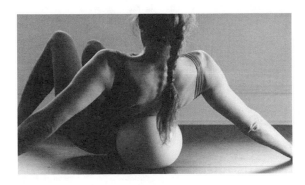

FIGURE 5.10

trapezius muscle fibers (figure 5.10), and then rolling the ball back to the next vertebra. At first it is difficult to isolate each thoracic vertebra, so start by working two or three at a time, rolling out toward the insertion of the lower trapezius at the inferior border of the spine of the scapula. Breathe as you roll the ball outward, expanding the ribs out toward the ball on the inhale and sinking into the ball on the exhale.

Change the angle slightly between T4 and T1 to follow the line toward the insertion of the middle trapezius on the superior border of the spine of the scapula. At T1, still staying on the right side of the spine, begin rolling directly upward to the top of the occiput to release the origins of the upper division of the trapezius. Since it is quite difficult to differentiate each cervical vertebra, it is best to simply work toward creating length in the cervical spine.

Next you will work down from the occiput, releasing the upper division of the trapezius toward its insertions at the lateral one-third of the clavicle, the acromion process, and the scapular spine. Roll back down from the occiput along the right side of the cervical vertebrae (figure 5.11) until you come to the first three thoracic vertebrae. You can lift your hips to put more pressure on the ball and keep it from sliding. Roll the ball along the superior border of the spine of the scapula (figure 5.12), resting at the acromioclavicular joint. As you roll you can either let your head rest on the ball and then on the floor, or, if you can maintain your balance, support the back of your head or neck with your left hand. As you roll along the upper trapezius you also release the origin points of the levator scapula at the transverse processes of C1–C4 toward their insertion at the vertebral border of the scapula. Breathe into this area as you roll, holding the image of spreading the scapula, shoulder, and neck outward.

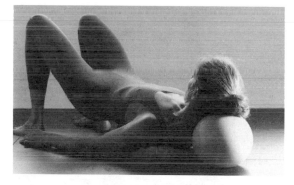

FIGURE 5.11

Once you have released the upper aspect of the trapezius out laterally to its insertion, roll the ball back in to the area between C7 and T5, the origin points of the minor and major rhomboids. After these origin points begin to release, roll the ball laterally and downward to the

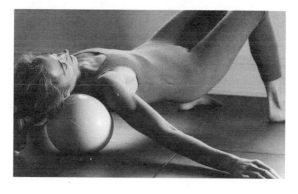

FIGURE 5.12

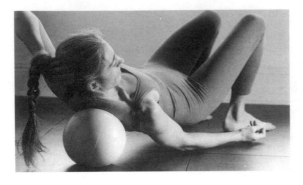

FIGURE 5.13

vertebral border of the scapula (figure 5.13), releasing the length of the rhomboids. With the release of the rhomboids, you have finished the right side.

Slowly take the ball away and lie on your back. Take a couple of deep inhalations and long exhalations and notice any changes in the right side. Feel whether this side is flatter on the floor than the left side. Can you breathe more fully into the right side than the left side? Does this side feel longer or more open?

Now repeat this same routine on the left side. As you work the left side, begin paying attention to the differences between the two sides, asking yourself how specific muscles on the left side feel in comparison to the same muscles on the right. Notice your coordination, flexibility, and sensitivity on each side. Making these comparisons is the way to develop the ability to perceive subtle differences in how you hold tension on the two sides and how they function differently in your day-to-day activities—an awareness you would not have if you only rolled up the center of the spine. Since the basic tool for solving body problems is awareness of sensation, the more developed your awareness, the more empowered you will be in your self-healing.

UP THE CENTER OF THE SPINE

Begin by placing the ball at the point between the ischium and the coccyx and gently roll it to the tip of the coccyx. The tip of the coccyx is often difficult to find; it can be easily broken or displaced to one side through a fall or a blow. If you cannot locate the coccyx exactly, place the ball in its general location. It is very important not to put all of your weight directly down on the coccyx; I have known people who became so enthusiastic about Body Rolling and spent so much time rolling with their full body weight on the tip of the coccyx that the coccyx began to turn under. Let your hands and feet take some of the weight.

As you begin to roll up the coccyx to the sacrum, make sure you spend time at each point. Staying in the center of the sacrum, deeply inhale, exhale, and sink, so that the maximum change can occur. You are going now for a change in quality of bone; if you roll up the sacrum too quickly, you will lose the momentum of the release you are initiating. Slowly and deliberately wait and breathe at each point of the sacrum.

It is also important to take time because you are working here not just structurally but on the energetic level. When you sit at the tip of the coccyx, you are waking up the point at the base of the spine where the kundalini energy enters. Another reason not to put too much weight on this point is that the weight would prevent the energy from flowing upward. If you do not open up this entry point, you will not achieve the deep level of relaxation described in chapter 3.

As you sit and breathe at each point on the sacrum, your breathing deepens and you begin to feel a relaxing sensation coming from the point where the ball rests. In fact, the longer you stay at any point, the more you can feel a release all around the spot where the ball is pressing. You can sense your legs, your pelvis, and your gluteus muscles all letting go, just from that continuous pressure on the sacrum.

When you finally get to the top of the sacrum, stay there a few moments. Then slowly begin to let the sacrum drop down over the curve of the ball (figure 5.14), creating a separation between the sacrum and the lumbar spine. You might want to hold the ball with your hands here, pressing it into the sacrum to keep

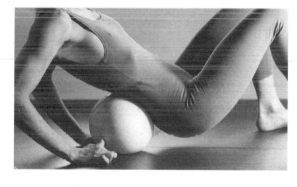

FIGURE 5.14

it from slipping. Continue to roll up the lumbar vertebrae, waiting at each point and breathing into the spot where the ball presses into the vertebra. Your focus is on creating intervertebral space between the vertebra you are pressing up against and the one below it.

Each time you move the ball up to the next vertebra, lift your pelvis slightly off the ground, curling it upward (figure 5.15). This motion puts more direct pressure on the ball, pushing it up into the next vertebra, and helps elongate the lumbar spine, flattening it on the floor. As you lower your pelvis back onto the floor, you can feel the vertebra you were just pressing on slide down. At first you might not be able to separate the individual vertebrae, so visualize the separation. As you continue to do this routine, the

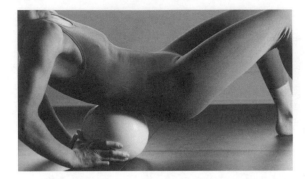

FIGURE 5.15

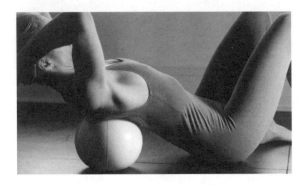

FIGURE 5.16

erector spinae muscles begin to release their tight hold on the spine, and you will be able to get that specific. Since the lumbar vertebrae are the largest in the spine, and most spinal flexion and extension comes from this area, the lumbar region is the easiest part of the spine in which to differentiate individual vertebrae. Once this area is released, you can work on separating the thoracic vertebrae.

This routine should be deeply pleasurable. If you feel any pressure in your head or neck, use one or both hands to support the back of your head (figure 5.16), keeping your neck long and your chin forward toward your chest.

Continue rolling up the spine, each time pushing the ball upward to the next vertebra by slightly elevating the pelvis, curling it upward to stretch the lumbar vertebrae and then relaxing down, putting pressure on the vertebra you are working. As you roll through the thoracic region, encourage the lumbar vertebrae to lie completely flat on the ground. Each time you drop a vertebra down, ask yourself: "Can I bring more of my back to lie flat on the ground?"

When you get to T1, stretch your neck out as long as you can and rest it over the ball (figure 5.17), feeling completely supported in the back of the neck. Bring your

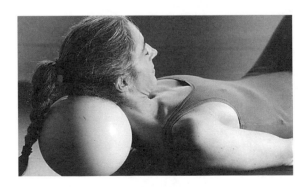

FIGURE 5.17

arms down to your sides. As you continue rolling, try to bring the upper thoracic vertebrae down away from the cervical vertebrae to lie flat on the floor. Bring your shoulders down to the floor, away from your head and neck.

It is even harder to feel the individual vertebrae and the creation of intervertebral space in the cervical region. Work slowly up the neck until you reach the top of the occiput, always visualizing that you are separating each cervical vertebra and bringing it downward from the ball to lie long and flat on the floor. Support the ball with one hand so that it does not slip out from under you.

Finally, hold the ball at the highest point on the occiput, where the occipital bone articulates with the sagittal suture (figure 5.18). Stay here for a minute or so, feeling for the greatest release possible through the back of the neck. Work your shoulders down to the floor, away from your head. Creating this maximum traction through the neck releases the trapezius, levator scapula, splenius capitus, and splenius cervicis muscles. Note that when you provide this space in the neck, these muscles release *on their own*. Transferring this insight to your practice means that, rather than putting direct pressure on these muscles, you can instead use traction to create space for them to elongate into.

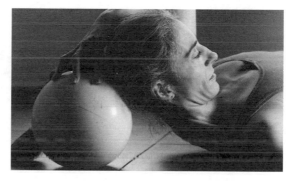

FIGURE 5.18

Support the back of the neck with one hand while the other hand takes the ball away, then slowly lower your head to the floor, rest, and relax. Take a couple of deep inhalations with long exhalations. Feel how your spine is lying on the floor. Is your back flatter? How is your breathing—does it flow more fully through your whole torso?

The lesson of this routine is that giving length is what enables muscle to release. The next time someone comes to you with neck pain, instead of pressing directly into it or just massaging the area of complaint, try giving length to the involved muscles and see if you achieve quicker and more effective results.

Giving the Back Routine to Clients

Lower back problems, so common in our culture, are a general category of complaint often treated by body-therapy practitioners. Thus, the basic back routines are the ones you will most often recommend to clients. In general, you want to convey the principle that no matter what the problem area, the goal is to create as much space there as possible. To give clients a goal to work toward, tell them that they want to achieve an elongated back, with long, strong, toned muscles that will support the spine and allow it maximum movement without pain or restriction. Explain that the ball provides both traction and focus for the mind.

The basic back routines are safe for everyone to use in keeping the back healthy and pain-free. When people claim they don't have enough time for the entire routine, give them only the instructions for rolling up the center of the spine. If you show them how to create the mood of working slowly and using the breath and the weight of the body to create space between vertebrae, they can do this routine in just fifteen minutes and still achieve a deep release.

UP THE CENTER OF THE SPINE

The following description exemplifies the amount of information needed to guide clients through the basic routine up the center of the spine. In actually presenting this routine you will need to keep reminding them to wait at each point, breathing and visualizing the vertebrae separating. Remember to speak slowly in order to establish a mood of relaxation and letting go. To help people create intervertebral space, give an image such as: "Now, letting your body weight sink into the ball at the center of each vertebra, breathe deeply into this point and visualize the muscles loosening their grip on the vertebra and releasing outward in all directions." This image gets people to focus at this small spot on each vertebra, demonstrating how you can begin to give them more detailed explorations. However, make sure the person you are working with first feels a more general sense of increased openness or lightness before she tries to sense more specifically for greater intervertebral space.

Sit on the ball and slide to the right so that you are resting on the right sitzbone. The left leg remains bent. With your left hand, reach back and feel for the end of your spine, which is the tip of your coccyx. Slowly roll the ball to that point. Now, with both knees bent and both feet on the ground, place your hands behind you so that your hands and feet are taking some of the body's weight off your coccyx.

Slowly begin rolling up the sacrum, a pear-shaped bone that is the base of your spine, stopping at each point for a full breath. As you exhale, let your body weight drop against the ball. Roll upward in this manner until you reach the top of the sacrum. *At this point, explain that it is important to work toward the separation of the sacrum and lumbar spine, since this area is generally overused and is therefore a point of great tension.*

When you reach the top of the sacrum, use your hands to push the ball down against the sacrum, separating it from the lumbar spine. Continue to roll upward with the weight of the ball pressing against the lumbar spine, dropping the sacrum down around the ball toward the floor. Curl your pelvis upward as you roll toward each new point, in order to elongate the lumbar vertebrae. Wait at each point for a full breath before rolling to the next vertebra. If you cannot feel the vertebrae individually, roll the ball each time to what you imagine is the next vertebra while letting the previous one drop down toward the floor. To prevent any feeling of strain, support your head with your hands after you roll past the lumbar area.

When the ball reaches the neck, hold the ball with one hand, stretch your head up and forward with the other hand, and then stretch your neck back over the ball. Lower your arms to the floor and work your shoulders down toward the floor, away from your neck and head. Take extra time to roll up the neck—this is an area that stores a lot of daily tension.

Now roll up the occiput, the bone in the center of the back of the head, holding the ball with one hand so that it does not slip. Really feel all the tension of the day releasing from your neck. Finally, support the back of your head with one hand and take the ball away with the other. Slowly lower your head to the floor.

Relax for a minute or so and breathe, noting how the body, lying on the floor, feels different from when you started. Does it feel longer? Are you more relaxed? Which parts of the back are resting flat on the floor?

UP THE TWO SIDES OF THE SPINE

For a more complete back release, and to develop greater body awareness, you can give clients this routine. People are often afraid to put the ball near the spine; let them know that it is important to work as close to the spine as possible, holding the image of tracing upward from one vertebra to the next. Your client can finish by rolling up the center of the spine again, for a total workout of twenty to thirty minutes.

Begin by sitting with the ball under the right sitzbone. Roll the ball upward toward the bottom of the sacrum. Keeping the ball on the right side of the spine, continue to roll point by point upward along the sacrum on the right side. Each point should be about one-half inch from the previous one. The ball should be pressing in toward the spine rather than out toward the hip. Take one full breath at each point on the sacrum, sinking your weight into the ball on each exhalation.

When you roll off the top of the sacrum into the back, hold the ball with your hands and push it downward against the right sacrum and right hip, breathing into the spot where it presses into the lower back and visualizing that you are elongating this area. Now let go of the ball, angle it in toward the spine, and begin to roll it slowly upward. As you move to each point, curl your pelvis up toward the ceiling and lift your hips off the ground in order to stretch out the lumbar spine. As you settle into each point, bring your hips down to the floor and take a full breath.

Since you will probably not be able to feel the individual vertebrae at first, roll the ball up one to two inches at a time and stay at each point for a full breath. As you breathe, visualize that you are separating the vertebrae, and that the muscles along the spine are elongating. If at any point you feel any tension in the back of your neck, support your head with your hands at the back of your neck.

Continue working up the right side this way. Each time you roll up a notch, pull your head up, chin toward chest, to stretch the cervical spine. As you roll up to the next point, continue to curl the pelvis up, flatten the lumbar spine out on the floor, and then let the pelvis come back onto the ground. Take a deep breath, trying to expand the entire right side of the rib cage.

Once the ball reaches the upper back, bring the head forward with the chin on the chest, really stretching out the back of the neck, and then let the neck rest over the ball. Continue to curl the pelvis up as you roll to the next point while also working your shoulders down away from your head, keeping the ball on the right side of the neck. Roll to about midway up the back of the head, holding the ball with one hand so that it does not slip out from under you. Stay at this point for several breaths, breathing into the back of the neck and feeling all of the muscles there relaxing and the neck elongating. Finally, support the back of the head with one hand while taking the ball away with the other.

Lay your head on the ground. Rest and relax as you feel for differences between the two sides. Does the right side lie on the floor differently than the left side? How does your lower back feel? How does your right leg lie on the floor in comparison with your left leg? Breathe and relax. When you are ready, repeat this same routine on the left side.

6

BASIC
SIDE
ROUTINE

Most of the time, body-therapy practitioners work either the front of a person's body or the back of the body. When you work the side, however, you are working the front and back together, for a few key lateral muscles link the muscles of the posterior and anterior aspects of the body. The goal in Body Rolling is to create a torso as long and as balanced between posterior and anterior as possible. Only by working on the sides of the body can you achieve maximum length in both posterior and anterior muscle chains simultaneously.

In working the side, you start by releasing the pelvis downward, beginning with the tensor fasciae latae. Elongating this muscle will set off a release in the muscles just posterior to it—the gluteus medius and gluteus minimus—and anterosuperiorly in the internal and external obliques, rectus abdominis, iliacus, and transverse abdominis.

After releasing the ilium downward, you can begin to move up the torso. Creating length in the first muscle above the ilium, the transverse abdominis, will stimulate release anteriorly in the internal and external obliques and the rectus abdominis, and posteriorly in the quadratus lumborum, latissimus dorsi, and serratus posterior inferior.

The next connecting muscle is the serratus anterior, which continues the release of the latissimus dorsi at its origin points on the ribs and in the front releases the pectoralis muscles. Release of the latissimus dorsi sets off release of the teres major and the muscles of the shoulder girdle and elongates the triceps. Release of the pectoralis muscles releases the biceps and the coracobrachialis. When you work laterally in this way, with the arm extended over the head and the leg extended downward, all the muscles in these chains, both front and back, are being elongated to their maximum length.

It is important to educate people to see themselves not as a front and a back but as a single whole torso. In both exercise and in the movements of daily life, they need to think not just about the back or abdominal muscles alone but about using all the muscle groups of the torso together to perform every task. For example, if I am bending over to pick up something heavy, I need to be conscious that I am not only using my lower back muscles but am also engaging my abdominals by pulling them in toward the spine to help make my whole abdominal and pelvic region strong, so that it works as a unit.

Most people tend to overuse the back, resulting in a contraction of the back muscles, a state that makes it harder to engage the muscles of the front. This imbalance can cause lower back problems, back-of-the-neck problems, and restricted shoulders. The side routine given here will balance anterior and posterior by elongating and stretching the muscle chains of both front and back. Working along the side in this way also gives these muscle chains the information that they can work together. When someone massages you on the front of the body, you do not feel your back; when the back is massaged, you do not feel the front. The side routine enables you to feel both front and back at the same time.

This routine is one of the most effective ways to create space between the hips and the rib cage, the area where most lower back problems arise. It also gives people a real awareness of how much the position of the shoulder and its range of motion (or lack of range) are affected by general tightness from the hip through the shoulder. And it demonstrates the powerful connection between releasing the rib cage and relieving shoulder problems.

There is a tendency in the field of bodywork to narrow the focus on shoulder problems to the shoulder itself, rather than considering the shoulder in relation to the rest of the body. According to my theory of working muscles in their natural order, however, the shoulder actually begins in the hip. If the posterior or anterior muscle chains are contracted at any point, they will pull the shoulder downward. The logical beginning in treating shoulder problems is to work the muscles from the hips and pelvis upward.

The side routine is also useful for people who cannot tell whether they are really breathing into the ball or not. Working up the sides of the ribs gives them the sensation of the lungs expanding out into the ball as they inhale, and they can really feel the sinking of the rib cage as they exhale. Finally, this is the most effective routine for helping people develop awareness of differences between their two sides and enabling them to feel dramatic changes after working one side. It is the exercise that most often allows people to observe connections that they did not know existed in their bodies. Even those with absolutely no somatic awareness are astonished by the results of this routine—they can, for the first time, perceive the sensation of muscle release.

Self-Exploration for the Practitioner

Begin by lying on your right side, legs extended; your weight is on your right hand,

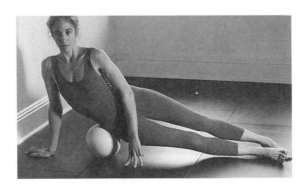

FIGURE 6.1

palm pressing into the floor with the arm straight. Your side is lifted and as long as possible. Place the ball at the top of the iliac crest along the origin of the tensor fasciae latae and begin rolling down the muscle toward its insertion in the iliotibial tract (figure 6.1). Roll as far as the head of the femur.

Now roll back up to the top of the iliac crest and try to stretch out the space between the hip and rib cage as much as possible. Press against the floor with your hand to maximize the side stretch, then roll the ball into that space (figure 6.2). Here you are rolling into the transverse abdominis and the internal and external obliques. Stay at this point and breathe into it, visualizing all these muscles releasing outward from the point of pressure. Feel the space increasing between the iliac crest and the ribs.

Extend your leg down long, out of the hip socket, and begin to roll the ball slowly upward to the lower margin of the rib cage (figure 6.3). Do not put any pressure on the floating ribs—they can break very easily. Instead, roll about three inches upward so that the ball is on rib eight or nine. The leg on the floor should be extended as long as possible. The other leg may be bent at the knee and placed in front or behind you to provide balance and support.

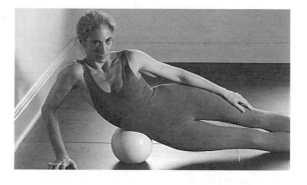

FIGURE 6.2

As you move up past the floating ribs, you stimulate release of the external oblique at its lower origin, around rib eight. Freeing the external oblique releases the ribs from the anteroinferior pull that a contraction in this muscle exerts on them. This release allows fuller expansion of the thoracic cage and enables you to focus more on the intercostals.

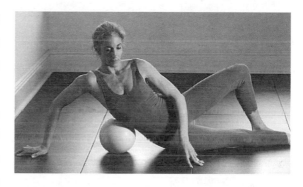

FIGURE 6.3

Beginning with rib eight, you will also be stimulating the release of the serratus anterior. On each rib from rib eight

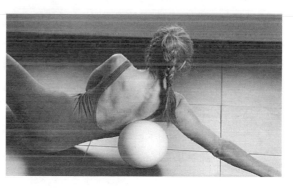

FIGURE 6.4

upward, roll posteriorly from the origin of this muscle on the rib along the muscle fibers to its insertion along the vertebral border of the scapula (figure 6.4). Continue to do this for as many ribs as you can up to the axilla. (Most people will not be able to access the origins on the first three ribs.) At each rib, concentrate on your inhalation, expanding the lungs outward to widen the rib cage and stretch the intercostal muscles.

As you roll through the length of the serratus anterior, you are also affecting the intercostals, key muscles of respiration. The internal intercostals run from the costal connection of the rib above posteroinferiorly to the upper border of the rib below. The external intercostals run anteroinferiorly to the upper border of the rib below, at a right angle to the internal intercostals. The ability of the intercostals to expand at different angles makes possible a 360-degree expansion of the rib cage. In order to get maximum movement in the rib cage you need as much intercostal space as possible; this freedom in the ribs then enables you to work for maximum length in the side. As you breathe, consciously focus on these muscles, stretching the ribs apart along their entire circumference on the inhalation, then contracting on the exhalation as the ribs come together and your weight sinks further into the ball.

Continue to roll, focusing on the inhalation. The work here is about using your inhalation to expand the intercostals from the inside out. Pressing against the ball helps you do this. If you feel any tension in your head or neck, bend the elbow of the right arm and rest your head on your hand.

The elongation of the side gives length to the longest muscle of the back, the latissimus dorsi. When the ball rolls between the iliac crest and the ribs and stimulates the transverse abdominis, it is also elongating the latissimus dorsi along its origin at the thoracolumbar aponeurosis from T7 to the iliac crest. As you roll up into the lower ribs, you are making a connection from the latissimus dorsi to the external obliques to the serratus anterior. Releasing these three muscles is what enables you to release a restricted rib cage. Further, without elongating the latissimus dorsi, you cannot release the muscles of the shoulder girdle: the teres major and minor, infraspinatus, subscapularis, and supraspinatus.

As you roll closer to the shoulder, extend your arm on the floor to elongate the latissimus dorsi out to its insertion at the bicipital groove of the humerus; let your head rest on your shoulder (figure 6.5). Most people never breathe into the upper one-third of their lungs and have little movement in the upper ribs. As a result, this part of the body is underdeveloped and inelastic. As the ball moves up further, use it to send air into the upper ribs and lungs by visualizing this area expanding as fully as at the lower border of the ribs, continuing the intercostal release.

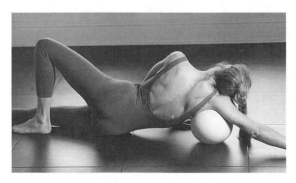

FIGURE 6.5

When you reach the shoulder, notice how the ball feels in your armpit. Can you feel your shoulder joint release, or does the ball meet resistance? To open the shoulder, bring the fingers of your left hand under the body of the pectoralis major (figure 6.6). As you pull the muscle gently away from you, roll the ball to the interior side of the muscle, push the ball medially, and breathe; letting the ball sink into this space where your hand is helps release the muscle more. Visualize elongating the pectoralis major from its origins on the clavicle, sternum, and costal cartilages of the upper six ribs out to its insertion at the lateral lip of the bicipital groove of the humerus. Let go of the muscle and roll the ball back into the axilla, putting pressure on the two origins of the biceps at the coracoid process of the scapula and the supraglenoid tubercle of the scapula. With your left hand, pull down on the body of the muscle in the direction of its insertion at the radial tuberosity (figure 6.7) as you visualize sinking the ball deeper into the origins.

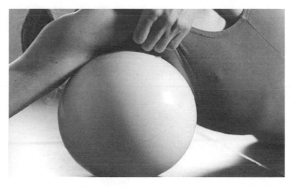

FIGURE 6.6

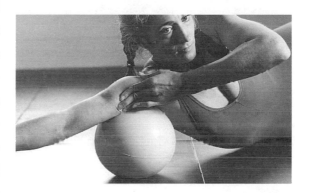

FIGURE 6.7

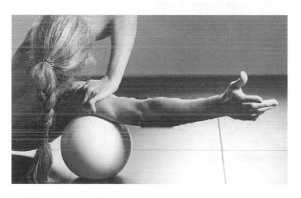

FIGURE 6.8

To work the triceps, reach around behind your shoulder with your left hand and grab the body of the muscle. Move the ball slightly posterior in the joint to exert pressure on the long head of the triceps, at the infraglenoid tubercle of the scapula, and on the lateral head, on the posterior humerus above the spiral groove. Extend the right arm out long, rotate it so the palm faces up, and with the left hand pull the body of the muscle down, toward its insertion at the olecranon process of the ulna (figure 6.8).

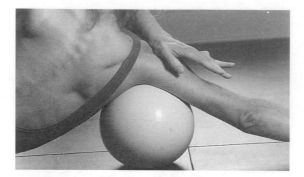

FIGURE 6.9

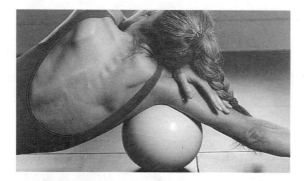

FIGURE 6.10

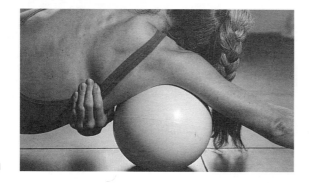

FIGURE 6.11

Then release the left hand and roll down the triceps to the deep head on the posteroinferior humerus.

Roll the ball back into the center of the axilla. Using the palm of your left hand, press downward from the origins of the deltoid (figure 6.9), on the spine and acromion of the scapula and the lateral one-third of the clavicle. Exert pressure both downward toward the ball and outward toward the insertion at the deltoid tuberosity. You can increase the pressure by laying your head on the back of your hand (figure 6.10). As you do this, visualize that you are creating space between the head of the humerus and the other bones that form the shoulder joint as you release the deltoid. When the deltoid is strongly contracted, it pulls the humerus up toward its origins, restricting range of motion of the humerus.

Now roll the ball slightly down the humerus. With your left hand, reach underneath the arm to find the inferior angle of the scapula; grab the latissimus dorsi and teres major between your thumb and fingers and squeeze (figure 6.11). Continue squeezing these muscles at the inferior angle of the scapula, trying to elongate them as much as possible and focusing the breath into the space between the ball and the left hand, visualizing the upper ribs expanding and the shoulder girdle opening. You are also giving maximum length to the serratus anterior, allowing it to release toward its insertion.

Finally, move the ball back into the axilla. Lying over the ball, notice the sensations around your shoulder girdle. Is the area more open than it was when you started? Is it easier to rest with the ball in your underarm? Does your right arm extend farther out on the floor? (In doing this routine, you may experience some numbness or nerve sensation in your hand or fingers. If this should happen, don't worry; these effects will be temporary. Sometimes when there is tightness in the muscles of the arms, direct pressure will stimulate nerves in an unfamiliar way.)

Before doing the second side, get up and slowly walk around the room feeling the differences between the two sides. Look at yourself in the mirror; the changes will be enormous. Note where you can feel and see changes: compare the two sides of your face and neck; notice differences in your shoulders; observe the expansion of the two sides of your rib cage; look for differences in the distance between pelvis and ribs on both sides. Knowing how many parts of you the side release affects can give you a lot of insight when treating clients.

After rolling up both sides, roll up the center of the spine as described in chapter 5. Because you have created additional length in the posterior and anterior muscles of the torso and the muscles of the rib cage, you need to make sure that the deeper erector spinae muscles take this same length. If the sides remain longer than the spine, the spinal muscles can cause the muscles just released to contract back to their original state.

Giving the Side Routine to Clients

It is important to explain to clients that we rarely feel the way the front and back can connect and work in harmony as we move. Working from the side with the goal of lengthening the whole torso, however, enables clients to feel this connection. You want your clients to understand that, as the ball rests at each point along the side of the body, it can be used as a focus to visualize expanding outward from that point both to the back and the front, while also lengthening from hip to shoulder.

Lie on your right side with the ball at your hip bone, stretching your legs out long on the floor. With the right arm stretched out and the palm pressing against the floor to support you, stretch your whole side as long as possible. Slowly roll the ball up from the hip to rest in between the hip and rib cage. The focus is on elongating the muscles of the lower back and lower abdomen. If you feel any pressure when the ball first touches the ribs, immediately move it up to the next higher point on the ribs.

It is very important to include this caution. Floating ribs can be very painful and, as noted earlier, they will break easily if they are rigid. Since clients will not know whether or not their ribs are rigid, it is better to cue them to move quickly upward if necessary, away from the area of the floating ribs. Since some people live by the "No pain, no gain" motto, you must tell them that this routine is not meant to be painful.

Slowly roll up the side of the rib cage, concentrating on your breathing, expanding your lungs and rib cage out toward the ball on the inhalation and sinking into the ball on the exhalation. At each point, visualize that the entire circumference of the rib cage is expanding. At the same time, imagine that on each inhalation your whole body is elongating from head to foot. Roll up to your armpit. When you reach your armpit, extend both your arm and leg as much as you can, working for maximum length of the entire side. Send your breath fully throughout your torso, visualizing that it is reaching every part of your back and front, from the hip to the shoulder. Try to imagine that your arm is actually moving up and out of your body; as you do this you can feel how the arm muscles connect to the body.

Before working the other side, lie on the floor and take a few deep breaths while sensing the differences between the right and left sides. Can you breathe more fully into the right side? Does this side feel longer? Slowly sit up, then stand and walk around, noticing the sensations in the right side. How has the work affected your neck, your jaw, your shoulder and hip?

Remind people that they should end this routine by rolling up the center of the back. The more they know about the body, the more you can describe specific muscles to work with in this routine.

CHAPTER

7

BASIC
FRONT
ROUTINE

Anyone who works remedially with backs knows that, in
order to have a healthy spine—and a healthy lower back, in particular—you need
strong abdominal muscles. However, most people strengthen the abdominals by doing
"crunches" and other contraction exercises, movements that contract the entire pelvic
area by shortening the abdominal muscles at their pelvic attachments. As a result of
these exercises, the latissimus dorsi, quadratus lumborum, psoas major and minor, and
iliacus muscles also become contracted. Contrary to this popular thinking, especially
prevalent in the fitness industry, I believe that healthy abdominal muscles are elongated, elastic, and strong. These three qualities define "well-toned" muscle.

The abdomen is the one area of the body in which enormous conscious effort is
required to maintain muscle length and tone. Almost all our daily activities—
especially sitting and sleeping, which take up a great many hours for most people—can
be performed without actively involving the abdominal muscles.

Everywhere else in the body, muscles run along bone, which helps the muscles to
maintain their length; however, the abdomen is an open cavity on which gravity and
the pressure of the internal organs exert a strong downward pull. As a result, the ribs

collapse and the abdominal muscles are pulled downward into the pelvic area. The goal of the Body Rolling abdominal work is to lift the abdominal muscles and visceral organs back up to take their proper place. The thoracic cage can then maintain an upright posture.

The basic front routine focuses on the rectus abdominis, the muscle with the greatest vertical length in the abdominal area. Working this muscle to its maximum length will also give greater length and function to the other abdominal muscles. (See chapter 9 for detailed work on these muscles.) Due to the weight of the organs dropping into the pubic area, where the muscles are weakest, the tendon at the origin of the rectus abdominis loses its elasticity and its memory of its lifting function. The goal of the front routine is to wake up this tendon and restore its lift.

The overlapping attachments of the diaphragm and psoas on the anterior spine comprise another important area affected by the front routine. When this area is severely contracted, it bends the body forward. This contraction will also compromise the function of the more external abdominal muscles, preventing the rectus abdominis from truly elongating. Most methods of stretching the superficial muscles will not release this powerful holding pattern; however, as you lengthen the rectus abdominis with the ball, you will initiate release and create length in this area as well.

Sometimes prolapsed or congested intestines exert pressure posteriorly, causing referred pain in the lower back. Such a problem may be resolved by treating the abdomen. Finally, the front routine promotes balance by helping the muscles of the anterior body work in harmony with the muscles of the posterior body to keep the posture as erect as possible.

Self-Exploration for the Practitioner

Come down onto your knees and elbows and place the ball on the pubic bone (figure 7.1). The knees can be as wide apart as is comfortable. Normally this point is not sensitive, although it can be uncomfortable for women before or during menstruation. If for any reason this point is painful, take additional weight on your knees and elbows.

Place as much pressure as possible on the pubic bone; stay there and breathe. The

longer you remain at this point, the more
strongly you will feel the connection
between the pubic bone and the sacrum.
The sacrum attaches to the pelvis via the
sacroiliac joints. Pressure on the pubic
bone therefore begins to release pressure
in the sacroiliac joints, creating an
extremely soothing feeling in the sacrum.
You can feel the joints beginning to
breathe more fully.

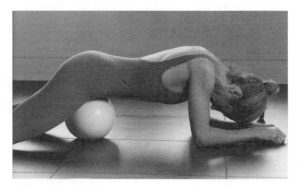

FIGURE 7.1

At this point, you are also applying
pressure to the origin of the rectus abdominis. As you bear weight upon this tendon it begins to wake up. Now slide off
the pubic bone into the abdominal area,
keeping part of the ball still on the pubic
bone and the other part on the abdomen

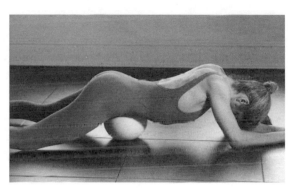

FIGURE 7.2

(figure 7.2). Stay there, focusing on breathing into the point where the tendon begins,
giving the tendon time to release with the intention of stretching it and restoring its
elasticity so it can release the rectus abdominis upward.

You are now intensely feeling the ball sinking in. As the tendon stretches, the
pubic bone actually drops down around the ball. This can be painful, so use your breath
to control any discomfort. As you inhale, push your belly out into the ball, and as you
exhale, sink into the ball. If the ball hurts as you sink, exhale less fully and inhale again
right away, pushing your belly out. At each exhalation, see if you can sink a little
deeper.

The longer you stay at this point and breathe, the more you will elongate the rectus abdominis. As the ball sinks now, it goes deeper into the belly. Meanwhile, you are
supporting yourself on your elbows and knees, which also helps control the amount of
weight you put on the ball.

After you have let the ball sink in as far as you comfortably can, roll it upward
point by point about three inches, into the center of the abdomen (figure 7.3). You are

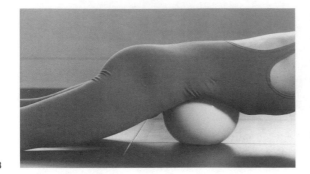

FIGURE 7.3

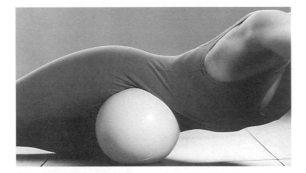

FIGURE 7.4

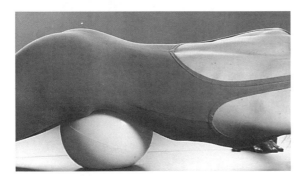

FIGURE 7.5

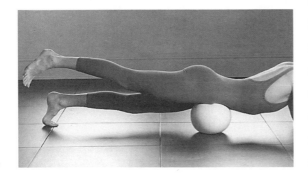

FIGURE 7.6

now stimulating the small intestines, which are commonly knotted up with tension that we unconsciously store there. You can release this internal tension by visualizing your breath filling up the tense area with air on the inhalation, giving the intestines more space, and then on the exhalation letting the ball press into the tight area to release it further.

Next, move the ball toward the right ilium, trying to insert it as deeply as possible into the inner surface of the bone and using it to push the ilium out laterally (figure 7.4). Your image is of scooping out the inside of the hip. You might want to shift your body to place more direct weight on that side (figure 7.5). Here the ball is releasing the internal and external oblique muscles and the origins of the deeper iliacus muscle on the inner surface of the ilium. Stay at this point and breathe.

Now raise your right leg off the ground a couple of inches, extending it straight out (figure 7.6). This movement starts to release the rectus femoris and sartorius muscles from their origins at the anterior inferior iliac spine, making you aware of their connection with the abdominal muscles. If the abdominal muscles are dropped into the pelvis, they can limit range of motion in these two leg muscles, which in turn affects the quadriceps and adductor muscle groups.

Bring the right leg back down to the floor and move the ball back to the center of the abdomen. Repeat this sequence on the left side, feeling for relationships between the two sides and for how this work on the abdominals might affect the back. Sometimes when working on the abdomen you might feel a discomfort you customarily notice in your back. This tells the mind that there is a connection between your back problem and the part of the abdomen you are working. As you raise the left leg, note which leg was easier to raise.

Roll back into the center of the abdomen and continue rolling up the rectus abdominis. Above the navel the work becomes a little more difficult, since you are moving into the area where the diaphragm and psoas muscles overlap at their origins, at the first three lumbar vertebrae. Since this is a key point for postural correction, it is important to work with your legs stretched out as long as possible and also to extend your arms above your head, stretching the other origins of the diaphragm at the lower six costal cartilages and the xiphoid process (figure 7.7). Stay there and breathe, focusing on expanding the rib cage upward on the inhalation while stretching the whole upper torso and the arms as long as possible. This is challenging, at first, for most people (and you may find yourself burping afterward). Thus, you do not want to remain in this position for too long—two to three rounds of breath is a good amount of time.

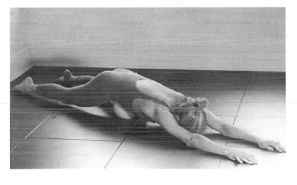

FIGURE 7.7

When practicing this part of the routine, it is important to focus your visualization on the origin points of the diaphragm and psoas at the first three lumbar vertebrae. Body-therapy students are often taught that deep muscles cannot be palpated, but if you visualize yourself sinking into this area you will get a release of the diaphragm upward—which frees the chest—and of the psoas downward. The separation of these two muscles releases the solar plexus. If you cannot actually palpate them, you can certainly affect them, especially if your intention is clearly focused.

Now lower your arms to rest on your elbows, and roll the ball up to the sternum

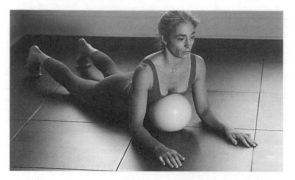

FIGURE 7.8

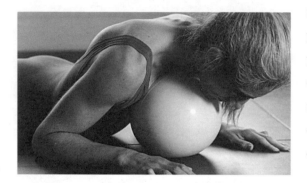

FIGURE 7.9

(figure 7.8). Do not rest the ball at the xiphoid process, which can be easily broken, but at the level where the sternum articulates with the seventh rib. Here, in the lung area, your focus is on the inhalation; having the ball on the sternum forces you to breathe into your back.

Try to feel the thoracic vertebrae corresponding to the level where the ball presses into the sternum. Putting direct pressure on this bone begins to release the costal cartilage, which in turn initiates release of the rib. This stimulates the other end of the rib at its vertebral connection.

Slowly roll up the sternum one-half inch at a time, waiting and breathing at each point and feeling for the connection to the thoracic vertebrae. Large-breasted women should use their hands to spread their breasts out to each side in order to keep the ball more directly on the sternum. (If you tend to have tender breasts before you menstruate, you might want to practice other Body Rolling routines at this time of the month.) Let your head drop down in front of you to put still more weight onto the sternum (figure 7.9). As the ball gets closer to the clavicle, lower your chin against the ball so that it does not pop out in front of you. The higher up you roll on the sternum, the tighter the contraction in the chest usually is, so you need to wait longer at each point for a sufficient release.

When you reach the clavicle, you begin to open up the front of the neck, elongating the scalene, sternocleidomastoid, and platysma muscles. Again, it can be challenging to breathe and wait here. People often cough at first, but as your muscles let go, you will be able to let the weight of your head and neck sink into the ball. This part of the routine also stimulates the anterior side of the cervical vertebrae.

Roll the ball up to the tip of the chin. Extend your arms forward to elongate the pectoralis major and minor and the latissimus dorsi muscles (figure 7.10), then try bringing them down by your sides (figure 7.11), stretching the sternocleidomastoid, scalene, platysma, and upper trapezius muscles. Now take the ball away with one hand. Lie on your back and experience your body.

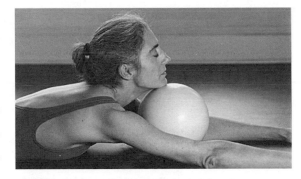

FIGURE 7.10

The front routine should be followed by rolling up the center of the back. When your time is limited, you can do just the front routine and then the back routine. But if you have more time, roll up the back, then up the front, then up the back again. You will see how much more release you achieve in the back the second time.

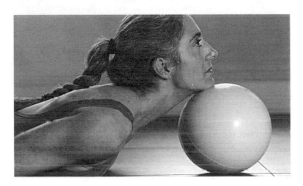

FIGURE 7.11

Giving the Front Routine to Clients

To help people do this routine most effectively, give them an image of increasing abdominal length and elasticity more and more at each point as they roll. They should understand that this routine affects the entire torso, so that as they focus on gaining length in the abdominal area, they are also elongating their back muscles out over the ball. Invite them to try to be conscious of activating muscles at each point in both the back and the front. The goal is to enable people to experience the feeling of energy rising through the body when they consciously work for length in the anterior torso.

With the ball pressing into your pubic bone and your elbows and knees taking additional weight, wait and breathe, trying to feel for connections between the pubic bone and sacrum. Then slowly roll off the pubic bone into the abdominal area, concentrating on pushing your belly out against the ball on the inhalation and sinking into it as much as you can during the exhalation. If this is too painful, inhale again and, rather than exhaling all the way out, exhale only partially and start inhaling again right away.

Roll up three inches from the pubic bone. Now gently roll the ball out to one side, pushing that hip outward, breathing into it and visualizing it opening outward. Roll over into the other hip and do the same. Then roll back to the center and continue rolling up the abdomen. When the ball rolls above the navel, you may begin to feel uncomfortable and find it hard to breathe. If so, move the ball to the bottom of the sternum without putting direct pressure on the tip of the sternum. If resting at this area of the abdomen is not too painful for you, stay here for a few breaths, making more space for the intestines to relax into, before moving up to the sternum.

Now roll very slowly up the sternum, waiting and breathing at each point, trying to feel whatever change may be induced by the pressure of the ball on the bone. Each time you inhale, think about opening up the point on the back at the same level as the ball is at on the front.

When the ball reaches the top of the sternum, see if you can stretch the front of your neck out and let it rest on top of the ball. Stay and breathe here, visualizing your throat softening as whatever tension you might be holding there releases. Now roll the ball slowly to the tip of the chin, stretching out the whole front of the neck. If it is too unpleasant to keep the ball against the throat, move the ball to the chin right away. Extend your arms out in front of you, observing how the extension affects the stretch in the neck. Now bring your arms down to your sides, pulling your shoulders down away from your neck and breathing into the front of the neck. Slowly release the ball and lie on your back.

Take a couple of deep inhalations with long exhalations. Has this work had any effect on your back? Has your breathing changed? Stand up and walk, noticing how your body feels.

Be sure to instruct your client to finish this routine by rolling up the center of the spine. Ask him to note how elongating the front of the body allows him to achieve a good release along the back as well.

PART THREE

More Focused Work

CHAPTER

8

LOWER
BACK
PAIN

In my experience, and according to most statistics, the majority of adults in the Western world experience lower back pain at some point in their lives. Certainly this is the complaint clients most often bring to body-therapy practitioners. People experience more "down time" from lower back pain than from any other type of structural problem. It not only inhibits people in athletic endeavors but constrains them in everyday life, as suddenly the basic movements we all do without thinking—getting out of a car or chair, or walking down the block—become enormous tasks.

People who suffer from back pain feel—consciously or unconsciously—that their bodies have let them down. Each wonders: "Am I going to be like this for the rest of my life?" The onset of back pain is often the first time that a person really appreciates all that the body does for us. Pain can be our best teacher, but only if we stop, listen to the messages it is giving us, and act on them.

I define the lower back as the entire lumbar spine, sacrum, coccyx, and pelvis, and all the muscles that have any attachments to any of those bones. Thus, to me the term *lower back pain* applies to any structural complaint in which pain is referred to any area in the lower part of the back and radiates down through the pelvis and legs.

The genesis of most lower back pain is overexertion, strain, poor posture, and, in general, chronic misalignment in the area of the body that takes the most weight. In treating lower back problems, therefore, the fundamental principle is to look closely at the client's general postural alignment and then consider what imbalances between different muscle groups have created that structural pattern. You then work the appropriate muscles to correct the alignment. This will balance the two sides of the back and pelvis and create space to relieve the pain.

It is not uncommon for people with lower back pain to do a great deal of exercise, yoga, or other practices they believe will help them, only to find themselves still in pain. The pain persists in part because they are doing these practices with the same faulty alignment that initiated the problem. Therefore you need to educate your client to understand the fundamental alignment problem so that she or he will not keep repeating the same pattern. With this approach you can both eliminate the problem and prevent it from recurring.

A weak, problematic lower back will always remain a vulnerable area, whether it hurts or not. Clients must therefore understand how to take care of the lower back on an ongoing basis, to keep it as healthy as possible. As a practitioner you must give people the information they need in order to work with their own particular problem.

Common structural reasons for lower back pain include collapse of the upper body; limited range of motion in the hips; misalignment of the pelvis in relation to the spine and legs; imbalances between various muscles in the legs, abdomen, and back; and imbalances between the front and the back of the body. The following muscle groups are involved in these misalignments:

- the muscle groups of the leg
- the abdominals
- the gluteus maximus, minimus, and medius
- the six deep lateral rotators
- the lower back muscles, including the latissimus dorsi, quadratus lumborum, posterior inferior serratus, and trapezius

The general principles for creating optimal space in the lower back are to work the leg muscles down from the hip, releasing them from their origins to relieve leg-related pressure on the hip; to work the abdominal muscles up from the pelvis; and to work the back muscles up from the sacrum.

Educational Routines for the Practitioner

I use these routines to teach practitioners all the muscles involved in lower back pain. Once you bring awareness to these muscles in your own body using the ball, you will begin to see interrelationships between them that will help you understand patterns and compensations in your clients' bodies.

POSTERIOR PELVIS ROUTINE

Begin by releasing the gluteus maximus. Place the ball at the origin points of the

muscle, along the posterior iliac crest and the posterior sacrum. Roll the ball outward toward its insertions at the gluteal tuberosity of the femur and the iliotibial tract (figure 8.1). Continue working down each origin point on the sacrum, each time moving toward the insertion; it is not necessary to roll all the way to the insertion.

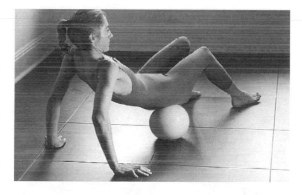

FIGURE 8.1

Now release the gluteus medius and the gluteus minimus. Place the ball superior to the iliac crest (figure 8.2) and roll down into the origin of the gluteus medius, on the ilium just below the iliac crest. Wait there, breathing and sinking into the ball. As the tendon releases you will sink down into the origin of the glu-

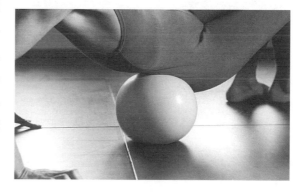

FIGURE 8.2

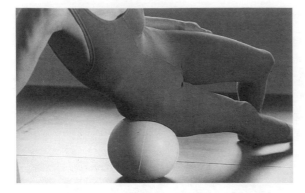

FIGURE 8.3

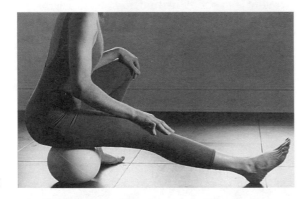

FIGURE 8.4

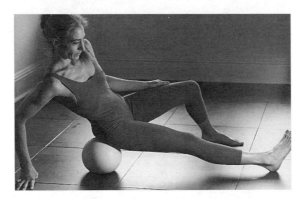

FIGURE 8.5

teus minimus, also on the ilium, below the orgin of the gluteus medius. You will feel it when you reach it—it is much shorter and tighter and more tender to roll through than the medius. Roll down to the greater trochanter of the femur (figure 8.3) and wait there, releasing the insertions of these two muscles.

From the greater trochanter, roll to the ischium; gently roll around the ischial tuberosity, the area where the three hamstring muscles originate. Slowly let the ball roll downward off the ischium; with the ball pressing on the ischium and just below it, again, wait and breathe. Here you are affecting the tendons of the hamstrings and beginning to release these muscles downward.

As you feel the tendons begin to release, very slowly roll four or five inches down into the hamstrings (figure 8.4), just enough so that the muscles get a sense of elongating down out of the hip. Roll the ball back up to the ischium. With all your weight pressing into the ball, visualize that you are tracing the pelvis from the ischium, along the ramus of the ischium, and to the acetabulum, over the path of the deep lateral rotators of the hip, from their origins on the ischium toward their insertions at the greater trochanter. At each point you can rotate the leg laterally and medially (figure 8.5).

This area can be very sensitive and so tight that it does not give. Wait and breathe at each point, in order to let the ball sink more deeply into these muscles. Because these lateral rotators are so deep, they can be difficult to work on with clients. The ball work helps you see other approaches and alternate leg positions to use in order to get at them.

Next, place the ball at the origin points of the tensor fasciae latae on the anterior superior iliac spine (figure 8.6) and wait, slowly sinking into this short muscle. Roll down toward its insertion in the iliotibial tract. Slowly continue rolling three to five inches downward into the iliotibial tract (figure 8.7). Then roll up to the hip, turn your belly toward the ball, place the ball at the origin of the sartorius in the notch between the anterior superior and anterior inferior iliac spines, and begin to roll inferiorly and medially (figure 8.8), following the muscle fibers of the sartorius, to about one-third of the way down the femur.

Now bring the ball to the origin of the rectus femoris, at the anterior inferior iliac spine. Roll inferiorly, along the rectus femoris, half-way down the femur (figure 8.9). Initiating length in the leg, the release of the sartorius is continued by the release of the rectus femoris, which allows easier access to the three deep vastus muscles. Contraction at the origins of the sartorius and the rectus femoris will pull the leg up into the pelvis.

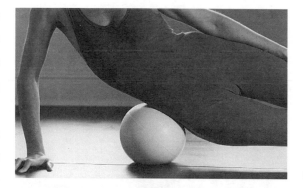

FIGURE 8.6

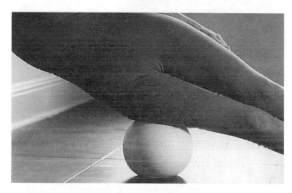

FIGURE 8.7

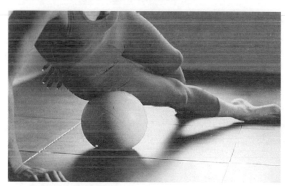

FIGURE 8.8

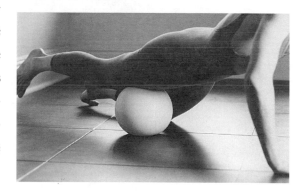

FIGURE 8.9

To release the vastus muscles, place the ball on the most superior point of the femoral shaft. Rotate your leg laterally and wait (figure 8.10). Then slowly roll medially. Return to center, roll down to the next point and again roll laterally, then medially. Repeat this procedure until you have rolled one-third of the way down the femoral shaft. This stimulates release of the vastus lateralis, intermedius, and medialis. These muscles can be virtually glued to the femur and to each other by connective tissue, a condition that inhibits the true function of each muscle. Wait at each point and breathe, with the weight of the leg on top of the ball, and visualize the muscles separating from each other.

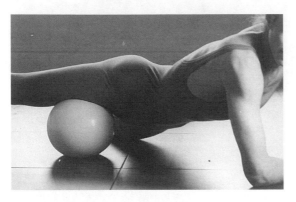

FIGURE 8.10

Now place the ball in your inner groin so that it presses into the pubis and pubic ramus (figure 8.11). The knee should be bent outward at a ninety-degree angle from the hip. Wait until the tendons of the adductors begin to release, then slowly roll the ball out to the medial knee. (For more detail on releasing the adductors, see chapter 10.)

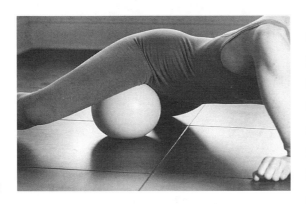

FIGURE 8.11

Repeat this routine on the other leg.

QUADRICEPS AND ABDOMINALS ROUTINE

To understand the connection between the quadriceps and the abdominals as a possible reason for lower back problems, do the basic front routine: roll into both hips, then up to the body of the sternum (see chapter 7). Next, follow the instructions in chapter 9 for rolling through the individual abdominal muscles—the rectus abdominis, the internal and external obliques, the psoas, iliacus, and transverse abdominis. Visualize lifting all these muscles up out of the lower abdomen. At the same time, visualize the muscles of the back elongating upward from the sacrum. As the quadratus lumborum relaxes its tight hold in the lumbar area, you can lift the rib cage up and away from the lumbar spine. As soon as this happens you can feel intervertebral separation, greater length in the lumbar spine, and release of tension held in the lower back.

Pay particular attention to the psoas major, an important muscle connecting abdominals, quadriceps, adductors, and the lower back. A contracted psoas will pull the quadriceps up toward the pelvis and the abdominals down into the pelvis, contract the quadratus lumborum, and inhibit the superficial abdominal muscles from taking their full length and tone. A short psoas acts as a strong internal lumbar lock that prevents the superficial muscles from keeping the anterior side of the torso elongated and upright.

LOWER BACK ROUTINE

Once you release all the leg and abdominal muscles that have any connections on the pelvis, you roll up the two sides of the spine as in the basic back routine, but this time with a specific focus. Your intention here is to eliminate any compression that might be causing discomfort. You have already released the muscles of the lower back; now the focus is to create length between the pelvis and the rib cage, using an image of creating as much intervertebral space as possible between S1, L5, L4, and up.

From being muscle-specific, you now shift to working on bone, focusing on separating each vertebra from those above and below and getting as much mobility in the spine as possible. By focusing on the individual vertebrae, you are also affecting the deep erector spinae muscles.

Routines to Give Clients

Clients with lower back problems can use the basic back routine for both sides of the spine as a good, safe, basic exercise to elongate all the back muscles and take pressure off the lower back. The two more specialized routines that follow are to be used as home maintenance for preventing and relieving lower back problems. Instruct your clients to finish each of these routines with the basic roll up the center of the spine.

Clients with spondylolysis and spondylolisthesis can do the basic back routine and the specialized routines, visualizing that they are getting the ball into the spaces between the vertebrae and lifting any vertebra that might have slipped onto the one below back into its natural position. The goal is to give space to the intervertebral disk.

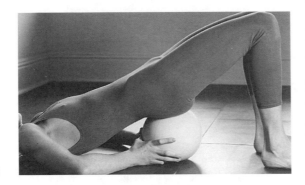

FIGURE 8.12

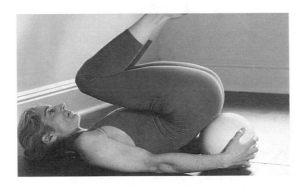

FIGURE 8.13

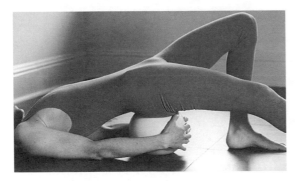

FIGURE 8.14

LOWER BACK ROUTINE #1

Lie on your back with your knees bent and your feet flat on the ground. Raise your pelvis and place the ball in the middle of your sacrum, holding the ball with your hands and pressing it into the sacrum (figure 8.12). Just being in this position begins to relieve the pressure in the lower back.

Inhale and raise your feet from the ground, bringing your bent knees up toward your chest (figure 8.13). You are now stretching out your lower back, which at the same time is being supported by the pressure of the ball. Breathe, expanding your lower back outward as you inhale, letting go and letting your weight sink into the ball as you exhale.

To come out of this position, exhale and very slowly bring your feet down, keeping the knees bent. This movement begins to strengthen the abdominal muscles. With the ball remaining under the sacrum, stretch one leg out on the floor as far as you can (figure 8.14). You will feel the quadriceps release, and you will feel the connection between the quadriceps and the abdominal muscles. Now stretch out the other leg.

Inhale, bringing the knees back up to the chest. With your hands, move the ball up a couple of vertebrae above the sacrum (figure 8.15). Keeping the knees at the chest, take deep inhalations and long exhalations, focusing the breath into the lower back. Use your hands to keep the ball pressing into the back. As you inhale, visualize the incoming breath making the lower back more spacious.

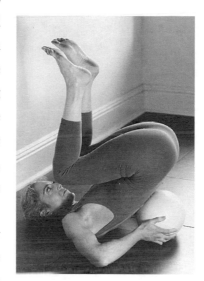

FIGURE 8.15

Continue raising and lowering your legs, bringing the feet to rest on the ground with knees bent. Each time you bring the knees back up to the chest, move the ball a little further up the spine. As you move your legs up and down, your lower back is completely supported as each vertebra is flexed and extended, increasing the general flexibility of the spine. Your image is of each vertebra moving both individually and also as a part of the whole spine.

Continue rolling the ball up your back as far as you can, while still keeping your shoulders and chest on the floor and bringing your legs down smoothly. Finish the routine at the point at which your shoulders or chest begin to rise or your movement in returning your legs begins to get jerky.

● LOWER BACK ROUTINE #2

People tend to think of a back problem as being *in* the back. They do not realize that there is an anterior side to the spine, and that often it is this side of the lumbar spine—where the psoas muscles have their origins—that is causing problems in the lower back. The following exercise is based on my theory that, in order to be strong, abdominal muscles must be long and toned. By giving length and elasticity to the psoas muscles, this routine integrates the two layers of abdominal muscles, enabling them to function in harmony.

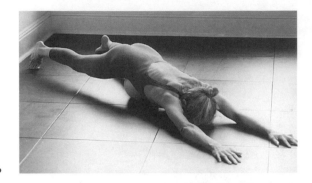

FIGURE 8.16

Place the ball at the pubic bone, as in the basic front routine (see chapter 7). Your focus is on how far you can sink the ball inward toward the front side of the spine. Straighten your legs and hold them at maximum extension, so your knees come off the floor and your legs are supported by your flexed toes (figure 8.16). Stretch your arms forward over your head, palms pressing into the floor. Your image is of a long, completely extended torso. Think: "As I stretch my abdominal muscles long, I am also stretching my back long."

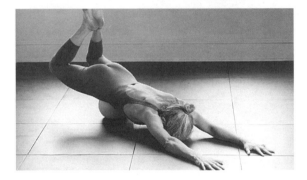

FIGURE 8.17

For those who can handle a slightly more advanced version, lift your knees off the ground without the support of the toes (figure 8.17). Hold this position for ten seconds, then exhale and let the knees down. Repeat ten times.

Clients with a true swayback should also imagine that, as the ball sinks into the abdomen, it is pushing outward against the front of the spine, elongating and flattening the curve of the swayback.

THE ABDOMEN
Postsurgical Conditions and Prolapsed Bladder, Intestines, and Uterus

When I ask people what part of the body they have the least awareness of and the least control over, most will say it is the abdomen. When I ask them to visualize this area, they think of a dark, unknown hole that contains the intestines and other viscera.

The abdomen is a soft cavity that the upper body naturally collapses into. Gravity also pulls the upper body earthward, putting extra weight on the pelvis and increasing abdominal pressure. The result is a tendency toward sluggishness in both muscles and organs, a condition that makes it difficult to maintain elongated, toned abdominal muscles.

A major function of the abdominal muscles is to keep the rib cage lifted, providing solid support and optimal space for the internal organs. The conventional wisdom about what makes the abdominal muscles strong and healthy is actually quite misleading. As I explained earlier, fitness-minded people, told to strengthen their abdominals in order to keep the lower back strong, do "crunches" and other exercises that keep these muscles tightly contracted. Yet any contraction of the abdominals contracts and shortens the space between the pelvis and rib cage and creates short, tight muscles in the lower back. Moreover, most people do their "crunches" with the abdomen pouching out, which means that the external muscles are pulling away from the psoas instead of pulling inward toward the spine to work with the psoas.

In the same way, when most people lift something heavy, they either let their abdominals hang relaxed or deliberately push them outward, putting a stress on the lower back. Neither slack abdominals nor tight abdominals can fulfill their enormously important function of supporting and moving the torso; this failure in turn affects the rest of the abdomen and the entire body.

Most people, except perhaps for those who have had an inguinal hernia, do not think of abdominal problems as being related to muscles. But if you think of the abdominal muscles as your clothing, the sheath that protects your vital organs, it becomes clear that if they are either too tight or too slack, they can affect organ function. Since the abdominals support the internal organs, when these muscles are collapsed and sluggish it is a strong indication that the organs are too.

For example, if the abdominal muscles lack tone, the intestines will not receive adequate stimulation; consequently, peristalsis will be sluggish. If slack abdominals fail to provide adequate support, there is a good chance that gynecological or urinary problems will develop, which with age can lead to a prolapsed bladder, uterus, or colon. Stress due to added pressure in the pelvis commonly leads to weakness in the abdominal wall and can result in an inguinal hernia. Even though much abdominal pain is not muscular in origin, properly functioning abdominal muscles can help relieve organ problems by giving the organs the space they need to function.

What these muscles need, then, is to be lifted away from the pelvic area and elongated up to their attachments on the rib cage to create maximum length in the abdomen. Once that general length is restored, it is important to develop maximum length, tone, and elasticity in the individual abdominal muscles. This combination is what accomplishes the goal everyone—body educators and fitness instructors alike—should aspire toward in their teaching: strong, long abdominals that take pressure out of the lower back and maintain the balance between front and back that keeps the torso strong, supported, and flexible.

Since most people have little instinctive awareness of the abdomen, we need to bring a whole new awareness to this part of the body so that the function of the abdominal muscles is recognized. The routines that follow integrate the different layers of abdominal muscles, so that the more superficial muscles learn to contract in toward the spine to work with the psoas.

Body Rolling abdominal work also differentiates the abdominal muscles from each other, in order to restore their function both separately and as a group. This is accomplished by working each muscle not only from origin to insertion but also from insertion to origin. This bidirectional work in the abdominal area is necessary because many of the muscle fibers cross and interlayer, making them likely to adhere to each other, particularly following surgery.

It takes a long time to restore neuromuscular function in the severed muscle fibers following any type of abdominal surgery, whether in the lower or the upper abdomen. When muscle is severed it loses its muscle memory; that is, it no longer understands its function. Muscle memory cannot always be restored. Deep layers of scar tissue often form after abdominal surgery, with adhesions between the layers of skin, muscle, connective tissue, and organs. If these adhesions are not broken up, a muscle may be unable to distinguish itself from all the other muscles, or it may be restricted or prevented from regaining its natural function. Working with the intention of giving each muscle its individual freedom of movement and length restores muscle memory and can break up scar tissue.

Educational Routines for the Practitioner

Releasing, separating out, elongating, and toning each abdominal muscle strengthens and tones the whole torso, increasing range of motion and relieving most hip and lower back problems. The following routines take you through the main muscles of the abdominal group. As you work each muscle from origin to insertion and vice versa, you will see how their overlapping and interweaving keep them very strong as a group. Once you experience the effects of taking each muscle to its maximum length, you will more fully understand the role that muscle plays in keeping the torso upright and free-moving. You will then have an incentive to maintain long, strong abdominals.

In these routines your focus should be on intensively visualizing each muscle, giving each one its greatest length from its origin, and freeing that muscle from the other muscles surrounding it. Working in such a way will give you a true, experiential sense of how each abdominal muscle contributes to making your torso as upright, strong, and toned as possible. Once you experience your abdominal muscles individually, you can work toward separating and differentiating each of these muscles in your practice, with the goal of creating a separation between the pelvis and upper body. As I lead people through this routine they can both see and experience the individual abdominal muscles, which become more defined.

Working these muscles also gives space to the diaphragm, which is important for maintaining length between the rib cage and the pelvis. I do not, however, recommend working directly on the origin points of the diaphragm with the ball. Unless they have worked to create considerable elongation of the abdominal muscles, in most people the area of the anteroinferior border of the rib cage is so rigid and contracted that they can hurt themselves by putting direct pressure there. Therefore, no routines specific to the diaphragm are presented in this book.

In exploring this routine it is important to follow the order given here, working from the most superficial to the deepest muscles. This sequence releases the more external muscle layers enough to enable you to access the deepest ones. Use an eight- to ten-inch ball, except where noted.

RECTUS ABDOMINIS ROUTINE

The rectus abodominis muscle, which gives the torso its greatest vertical length, is the easiest muscle to focus on when you want to keep your torso elongated. If you hold a clear visualization of this muscle in its full length, you can stay conscious of it during the day and keep it lifted. A long, toned rectus abdominis takes pressure off the pelvis and frees the adductors and quadriceps.

Place the ball low on the pubic bone, just below the origin of the rectus abdominis (figure 9.1). Wait and breathe, then slowly roll onto the point of origin. Stay there, allowing the tendon to begin to release, then roll slightly upward and to the right of center, so that the ball is partly on the bone and partly on the tendon as it extends superiorly into the abdomen (figure 9.2). Let the tendon continue to release, working to extend your legs as far away from your body as possible. Slowly roll through the tendon into the abdomen, visualizing releasing the muscle to its greatest length upward from the origin. Keep the legs long; this helps increase the length of the muscle.

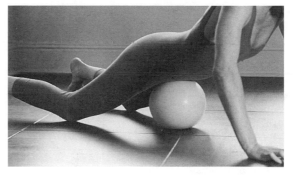

FIGURE 9.1

Concentrate on this origin point, trying to restore the elasticity at this lowest part of the muscle. Spending time at this point to stimulate the tendon is crucial, since this is the part of the rectus abdominis that most easily loses its memory because of the downward pull exerted by gravity and upper body weight.

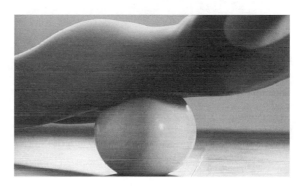

FIGURE 9.2

Now, extending your arms above your head, roll upward point by point toward the sternum (figure 9.3). Roll quickly over the diaphragm, as this is a tender area; continue rolling until the ball is on

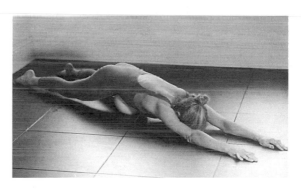

FIGURE 9.3

the sternum, about two inches above the xiphoid process. Be sure not to put pressure on the xiphoid process itself. Wait here and breathe.

Roll off the sternum to the right, onto the insertion point of the rectus abdominis on costal cartilage five (figure 9.4). Roll downward, following the line of the muscle fibers, to a point just below the diaphragm. Repeat this procedure from the insertions at cartilages six and seven, visualizing that the ribs are separating out from the sternum and that the sternum can lift upward out of the abdominal cavity. If there is a downward contraction at these insertion points, both sides of the rib cage will narrow toward the

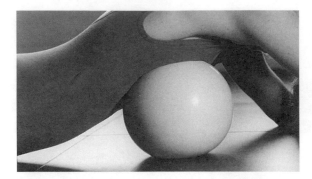

FIGURE 9.4

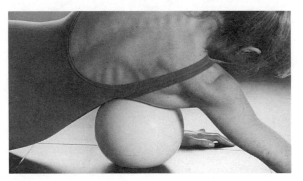

FIGURE 9.5

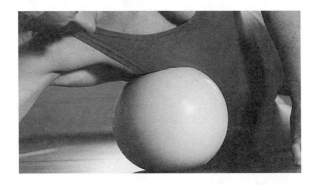

FIGURE 9.6

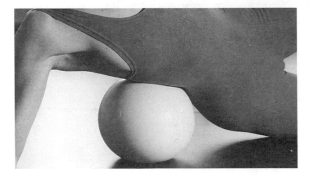

FIGURE 9.7

sternum, compromising the function of the diaphragm and the upper digestive tract. In my experience, everyone with upper gastrointestinal problems is contracted at the insertions of the rectus abdominis.

Follow this procedure on the left side. Finally, lie on your back and feel how this routine has affected your breathing, the way your back rests on the floor, the expansion of your ribs, and the length in your abdominals.

EXTERNAL OBLIQUE ROUTINE

The external oblique has its origins on the outer surfaces of the lower eight ribs and runs anteroinferiorly to insert at the abdominal aponeurosis and the iliac crest. Its fibers interlace with those of the serratus anterior and the latissimus dorsi.

Place the ball on the right side, at the highest origin point of this muscle (figure 9.5). Roll along the line of the muscle fibers in toward the center line (figure 9.6), breathing at each point. Roll back to the ribs and continue releasing this muscle from each origin point, rolling anteroinferiorly toward the linea alba. From the last three ribs, roll down to the insertion at the iliac crest (figure 9.7).

Wait here, breathing into the spot

where the ball is. Now slowly roll the ball
along the iliac crest toward the pubic bone
(figure 9.8), moving it from point to point
in micromovements. Visualize the muscle
fibers being stimulated and lengthened
toward their insertion. Try keeping the
right arm and leg extended. As you do this
routine, you can feel the muscle fibers of
the external oblique separating from the
other abdominal muscles.

Repeat on the left side.

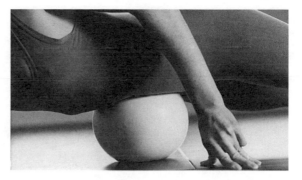

FIGURE 9.8

INTERNAL OBLIQUE ROUTINE

The internal oblique originates on the
inguinal ligament and anterior iliac crest
and inserts on the costal cartilages of the
last four ribs and on the abdominal aponeurosis. Toned internal and external obliques
support and contain the abdominal viscera,
keep the rib cage aligned with the pelvis,
and give length to the lumbar spine.

Use a six- or eight-inch ball for this routine.

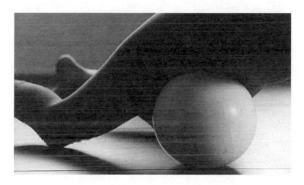

FIGURE 9.9

Place the ball on the right side of the pubic
bone, at the lowest origin point of the internal oblique along the inguinal ligament (figure 9.9). Roll slowly laterally and upward to
the highest origin point at the anterior iliac
crest (figure 9.10). From here, roll upward to
the muscle's insertion on the costal cartilage
of the twelfth rib (figure 9.11). Then bring

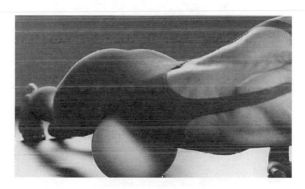

FIGURE 9.10

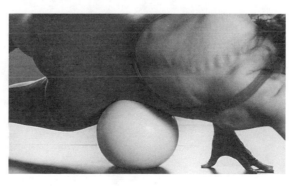

FIGURE 9.11

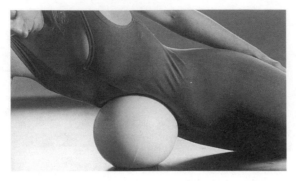

FIGURE 9.12

the ball back to the anterior iliac crest and move anteriorly to the next origin point. Continue to roll from the origin points on the iliac crest out to the insertions on the eleventh to eighth ribs.

Roll down to the next origin point on the iliac crest. Now roll medially to the highest point of the abdominal aponeurosis, just below the sternum (figure 9.12). Bring the ball back down to the iliac crest and continue working from each origin point, following the muscle fibers in to the midline until you reach the pubic bone again. Repeat on the left side.

TRANSVERSE ABDOMINIS ROUTINE

This deep muscle exerts a powerful holding effect, acting like a girdle that binds together the upper and lower body. Contraction of the transverse abdominis shortens the lumbar spine. Releasing this muscle is crucial for creating length in the lower back and in the torso as a whole, and for preventing lower back injuries.

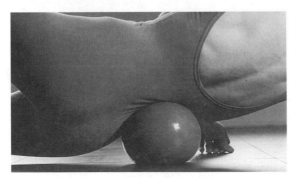

FIGURE 9.13

For this exploration, use a six-inch ball.

Place the ball on the right side of the pubic bone and roll toward the inguinal ligament. Trace around the iliac crest, rolling posteriorly between the iliac crest and the lower margin of the rib cage (figure 9.13). Roll into the thoracolumbar aponeurosis (figure 9.14), visualizing that you are pushing it in toward the spine. This action affects the origins of the

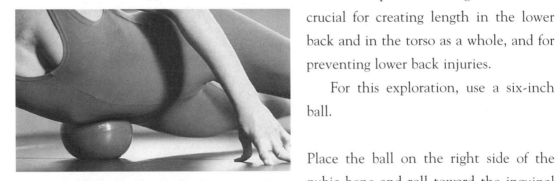

FIGURE 9.14

transverse abdominis both on the anterior iliac crest and on the inner edges of ribs six through twelve. This is the deepest abdominal muscle; to affect it you need to visual-ize sinking into the ball as deeply as you can at each point, while waiting and breathing. Also, visualize lifting your ribs up away from your pelvis and working your pelvis down away from your ribs.

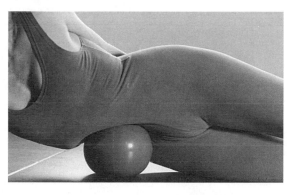

FIGURE 9.15

From the thoracolumbar aponeurosis, begin to roll directly anteriorly toward the central insertion point of the transverse abdominis, on the linea alba (figure 9.15). As you roll, visualize this muscle as an elastic band that, as it widens, releases the torso both upward and downward, allowing the thorax and pelvis to separate.

ILIACUS ROUTINE

The origin of this muscle blankets the entire inner surface of the ilium; it inserts at the lesser trochanter of the femur. When the iliacus is contracted, it contracts the adduc-tors, pulling the leg medially and superiorly and restricting range of motion as well as tightening the gluteus medius and minimus and the deep lateral rotators of the hip. Extreme contraction of these muscles can greatly restrict hip motion, and in severe cases can result in the need for a hip replacement.

Again, use a small (six-inch) ball for this exploration.

Place the ball on the pubic bone, then roll off the pubic bone to the right, pushing the ball into your right hip (figure 9.16), intending to affect the inside of the ilium. The transverse abdominis and internal and external oblique muscles can all become attached by connective tissue to the iliacus, so as you do this movement

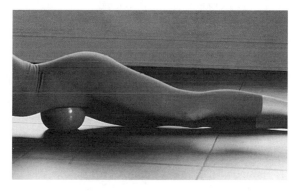

FIGURE 9.16

visualize these muscles separating from the iliacus, freeing the iliacus so that it can release at its insertion and free the femur. Creating this separation frees the abdominal

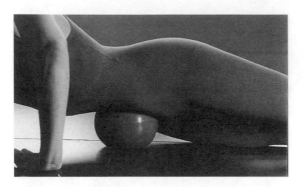

muscles from involvement with problems in the hip joint. Extend your right leg and rotate it medially and laterally to stimulate the insertion of the iliacus at the lesser trochanter.

Shift your weight to the left to push the ball farther into your right ilium (figure 9.17). Your left hand is on the floor, lifting your body so as to apply more weight to the ball. Wait, breathe, and feel the ball sink in. Note that just applying pressure into the anterior side of the hip enables you to feel the muscle's insertion point in the leg.

PSOAS MAJOR ROUTINE

The psoas major, which originates from the bodies of T12–L5, is the primary hip flexor and is also the muscle responsible for maintaining free movement between the pelvis and legs. When the psoas major is tightly contracted, the other abdominal muscles cannot achieve their greatest length, and consequently the torso will be unable to assume a full upright position. The abdominal organs will thus be unsupported and may prolapse. A contracted psoas may also cause a strong lordosis.

Use an eight- or ten-inch ball initially for this routine; after a while you can switch to a six-inch ball, which provides a more intense experience.

Begin with the ball at the pubic bone. Roll the ball off the bone and up toward the abdomen. Extend your legs, wait, and breathe, seeing how far into the abdomen you can sink the ball. Visualize that you are sinking the ball toward the spine. When you have sunk as deep as possible, stay at that depth and roll up the center of the abdomen until the ball is approximately level with the navel (figure 9.18). Extend both arms and legs, working for length and trying to sink in farther to reach the anterior spine. You are now at T12–L1, the highest origin point of the psoas.

Shift the ball so that it is on the right side of the anterior spine (figure 9.19); this pressure will affect the anterior right side of T12–L1. Slowly roll down toward the pubic bone, visualizing that you are working each lumbar vertebra from the anterior side. Extend the right leg as long as possible, turning it outward. This stimulates the insertion point of the psoas on the lesser trochanter.

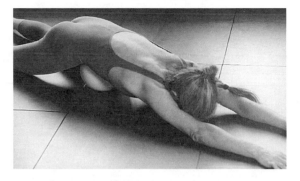

FIGURE 9.18

Now repeat the routine on the left side.

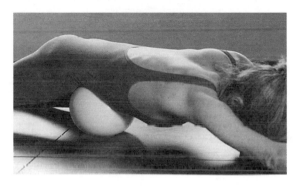

FIGURE 9.19

Since the psoas major is such a deep-lying muscle, as you work it is important to visualize the muscle very clearly in your mind, imagining that, as the ball rolls down past each origin point, that point is releasing down the lumbar spine to give the muscle more length. Simultaneously elongating the leg on that same side stimulates greater length at the insertion. You will notice a big difference between just knowing the location of the psoas major as a conceptual fact and really focusing on it almost as a meditation. Maintaining your focus and intention also helps you through the discomfort of working this deeply.

Routine to Correct Prolapses

The most common reason for prolapses of the uterus, bladder, or colon in women is childbirth. However, prolapses can also be caused in both men and women by severely collapsed abdominal musculature maintained over years. I believe that when an organ is prolapsed, its normal level of functioning is greatly inhibited. Even when its normal position has been lost, however, the correct position is still imprinted somewhere in the brain, and when the organ is repositioned where it belongs, it begins to function properly again.

To reposition a prolapsed organ, you need to educate the muscles that should be holding it in its natural position to restore their optimal length and tone. The general principle is that any prolapse must be lifted, whether you are lifting muscle alone or muscle and organs. The basic abdominal routine will do wonders for all prolapsed abdominal organs. Elongated, lifted muscles will hold these organs in their optimal position, restoring the space they have lost through gravity or other causes.

You can make the basic front routine more powerful by using the breath. Try the following technique, based on the yogic practice of *uddiyana* or "abdominal lift," and see how deep into the pelvic area you can go. This practice pulls the abdominal muscles up, restoring the muscle tone that will lift prolapsed organs. It is also tremendously helpful in releasing the psoas. Once you teach clients this technique using the ball, you can ask them to apply the abdominal lift when you are working on them. With the abdomen lifted in this way, you can feel each separate abdominal muscle and work it individually; you can also feel each individual organ. Using this technique also minimizes discomfort for clients unused to a body therapist working deeply in the abdomen.

Lie on the ball with your weight partly on the pubic bone and partly on the lower abdomen (figure 9.20), stimulating the origin of the rectus abdominis. Take a deep inhalation and a long exhalation. Now take another deep inhalation and blow all the air out of your mouth as forcefully as possible. Without breathing in again, pull your abdominal muscles in and up toward the rib cage as strongly as you can—you will feel the ball sink deeper into the pubic area. Stretch out your arms and legs.

When you need to breathe again, let go of the lock, relax your arms and legs, and take several full breaths, then try the technique again.

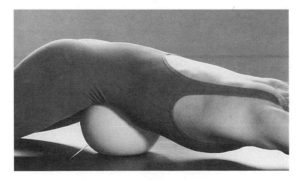

FIGURE 9.20

Postsurgical Routines

When the abdomen is cut all the layers of tissue contract, from the skin through the layers of muscle and connective tissue to the deepest internal organs, and their metabolic function is greatly reduced. All the muscles that have any connection to the area around the incision are affected. Often, for example, a lower abdominal incision will cause the quadriceps or adductors to shorten upward, restricting leg movement. As the healing of severed muscle begins, all the surrounding tissues contract toward the incision. As scar tissue develops, adhesions build up within the soft tissue; various tissues might also attach to organs and to the spine, further decreasing function. Following surgery, it is absolutely essential to break up scar tissue in order to restore optimal function on all levels.

The following routines restore tone to abdominal muscles faster than any other abdominal exercise. They will break up adhesions, begin to reconnect the cut ends of muscles, separate the different muscles that might have become attached to each other by connective tissue, and begin to restore muscle memory. Before doing them, wait until your physician has told you that the incision is completely healed and that you can resume a full abdominal-exercise program. (The usual time frame is six to eight weeks from the day stitches were removed.)

LOWER ABDOMINAL INCISIONS

For caesarean section, inguinal hernia, and appendectomy incisions, begin with the ball on the pubic bone, but do not put all your weight onto the ball (figure 9.21). Let your legs, elbows, and hands take the weight, increasing the pressure on the pubic bone slowly over time. Roll slowly upward toward the incision several times,

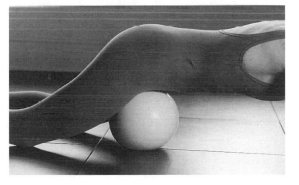

FIGURE 9.21

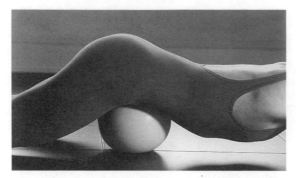

FIGURE 9.22

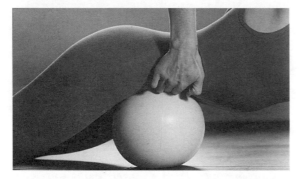

FIGURE 9.23

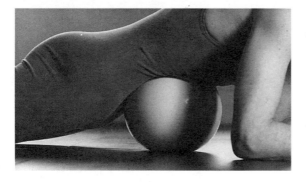

FIGURE 9.24

each time from a different angle. At the same time, slowly and carefully try to stretch your arms above your head and your legs away from the abdomen (figure 9.22), a little at a time. Work with the image of stretching everything up and away from the incision while the ball is beneath it. Next, to work with more detail, use your fingers to press and lift the abdomen upward, away from the incision (figure 9.23).

Now place the ball superior to the incision. This time, with the ball exerting traction upward, it is particularly important to stretch the lower part of your body downward (figure 9.24). Use your breathing here: As you inhale, really expand your abdomen outward, stretching the incision in all directions. Exhale and let the fibers relax back toward center. The main work occurs during the inhalation. Visualize spreading all your muscles, skin, and connective tissue free from their attachments to the incision, and imagine natural function returning to all your muscles, organs, and connective tissue.

Once you have gained some elasticity around the incision, you can roll directly up onto it. At each point, roll from below the incision, to directly on it, and then roll above it. Hold the image of pushing the whole incision out into the ball. As you inhale, visualize that you are expanding all the layers that have been cut into. As you exhale, let the ball sink through the incision, into as deep a layer as possible. Your body weight and the ball will break up the scar tissue.

● UPPER ABDOMINAL INCISIONS

To prevent rib cage contraction after gallbladder and other upper abdominal incisions, begin at the pubic area and roll the ball up the rectus abdominis. Then roll the ball upward from both iliac crests to just below the incision. Breathe at those points, stretching your arms overhead. Hold the image of lifting your rib cage as far up and out as possible from the incision, as you also work to elongate the abdominal area. You can use one hand to spread each side of the ribs as you breathe (figure 9.25).

If there is any downward pull of the ribs toward the incision, work the external obliques anteriorly downward from their origin points toward their insertion at the linea alba. Next, roll downward from the insertion points of the rectus abdominis to free up any medial contraction at the border of the ribs.

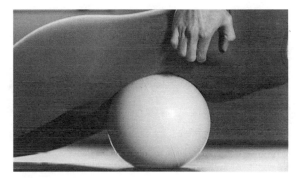

FIGURE 9.25

If there is a downward contraction of the internal obliques, work down from their insertions on the costal cartilages of the last four ribs, the arms stretched overhead. Breathe into the point where the ball is and visualize the rib cage expanding upward, the two halves of the rib cage separating away from the sternum.

Finally, after you have gained some elasticity in the tissues, place the ball directly along the incision. With your arms extended over your head and your legs outstretched, breathe at each point, pressing your abdomen out against the ball on the inhalations and sinking into the ball on the exhalations. Visualize the ball sinking through the layers of scar tissue and gently breaking up the remaining adhesions.

10

LEG, FOOT, AND ANKLE ALIGNMENT

Leg problems of any kind, whether affecting the muscle tissue or the bony structure, are always due to joint misalignment. A chronic misalignment in the hip, knee, or ankle will throw the entire leg out of balance. For this reason, any discussion of leg problems must begin by defining proper alignment.

When the femur is properly aligned in the acetabulum, all the muscle groups of the thigh are toned and free of restrictions. The joint has adequate lubrication and intra-articular space, and the femur moves freely in the hip socket, with no tight tendons restricting it.

This well-aligned hip places the knee directly in line below it, with the patella centered and resting superior to the femur-tibia articulation, and with adequate intra-articular space. A knee that is turned medially or laterally indicates an imbalance in at least two of the muscle groups of the thigh.

An optimally aligned ankle is directly in line with the knee and hip. There is space between the tibia and fibula and also between all the bones of the foot. The ankle has complete range of motion, meaning that as the foot rotates, it can reach each point of the circle equally without the knee moving from its neutral position. A knee that moves with the ankle indicates tightness of muscle between knee and ankle.

In the balanced leg, all three joints bear equal pressure. Any injury disrupts this balance by putting excess pressure on one or both of the uninjured joints. Usually, just the joint immediately above the injured one is initially involved. For example, since all the muscles that run down into the ankle have their origins at or just below the knee, a sprained ankle will affect the knee. If the ankle is treated right away, with the muscles released from the knee down to the ankle and the ankle worked in its entire range of motion, the sprain can usually be resolved quickly and the inflammation and swelling alleviated. If, however, the sprain goes untreated for a while, it will start to involve the hip as the injured person compensates for the pain in the ankle. When there has been a delay in treatment, therefore, you will need to treat the entire leg. In general, any problem anywhere along the leg must be treated by working at least two joints, and optimally all three.

Because we are never actually taught how to walk, most of us do so with little awareness. Small children learn to walk by experimenting; once they can balance, they simply continue in the same pattern as they began. Even adults rarely use their analytical capacities to investigate how they use their legs. Consequently, people take walking for granted and do not understand how connected the feet are to the rest of the body, or how the muscles of the legs and feet work to create these movements. Walking is produced by the thrust and momentum of all the leg muscles down into the feet and toes, and various factors can prevent these muscles from working properly.

Most people have one foot that is weaker than the other due to lazy muscles that allow the ankle to collapse into the foot. Others are born with flat feet or have weak and undeveloped foot muscles; those muscles never achieve their natural function unless they are specifically taught. In addition, most shoes—sneakers no less than high heels—cut off the thrust of the leg muscles at the foot. The muscles that run from the calf toward the toes are responsible for moving the foot and toes, and the way we place the foot down at the end of a movement is important. But when the foot is locked into a shoe, these movements cannot complete their thrust, cutting off the function of these muscles at their insertions. As a result, the foot muscles themselves are almost never used in walking or standing, and can atrophy even during an active lifetime.

In most cases, the way we walk and stand determines the alignment of the legs.

Someone who walks more heavily on the right side or bears more weight on the right leg when standing will often have what appears to be a shorter right leg, probably accompanied by a greatly decreased range of motion in the right hip and a stiffer right knee. These changes will then weaken the left leg and hip. The hips will be out of alignment, and over time the joints on the right side will lose intra-articular space and may begin to degenerate. Restriction in a hip joint can also contribute to a lower back problem.

Misalignments in the hips and knees solidify in the feet, causing calcification there much earlier than anywhere else in the body. This happens partly because the feet take all the faulty weight-bearing of a misalignment, partly because circulation decreases in the extremities more rapidly than elsewhere in the body, and partly because the muscles of the feet have lost their elasticity due to lack of use. As a result, any imbalance in the leg from hip to knee to foot, if maintained for a long period of time, will calcify the foot into a correspondingly distorted pattern.

People who walk heavily or do much high-impact exercise also often lose the natural shock absorption of the intra-articular space in the ankles, the space that keeps the bones from touching each other. (As a result, the tarsals, each of which should glide separately as the foot moves, become fused.) The decrease in space within the ankle forces the knee to absorb more weighted impact. If this extra stress persists over time, the knee can weaken and become injured, resulting in increasingly limited range of motion in the ankle. Most common knee injuries are caused by a wearing away of the menisci due to too much impact or other extreme stress on the joint.

Continuous impact on the knee gradually builds up intra-articular pressure. The cruciate ligaments and the menisci have increasingly less room, and lubrication of the joint diminishes. To restore the space, the bones must be separated. To do this you need to work not on muscle but on bone, with the specific intention of separating the tibia from the femur and the patella from both of these.

From the perspective of alignment, then, it is clear that the standard practices for developing strong leg muscles—deep knee bends, squats, and steps—can be counterproductive. They only inflict more pounding and stress on the leg joints, exacerbating whatever misalignments may already exist. Instead, strong and well-toned muscles can be achieved by freeing each muscle in the leg, giving each one its full length and ability to function, not only with the other muscles of its group but also individually. One goal of the Body Rolling leg routines is to separate the thigh muscles, which tend to adhere to the bone or to each other, restricting movement of the femur and decreasing circulation. The goal is a longer, streamlined leg in which the muscles have their proper length and freedom of movement. There is then less weight and pressure bearing down into the feet and circulation increases, diminishing the risk of developing congestive conditions such as cellulite, varicose veins, and joint problems.

In treating legs, therefore, I have two objectives: to release muscles and to separate bones. Freeing all the muscles is necessary for creating space in the joints. Separating bones relieves intra-articular pressure that has built up over years.

This chapter does not discuss specific injuries, for I believe that using Body Rolling to create length and balance in all the muscle groups of the leg both addresses and will prevent a multitude of possible injuries. If a client comes in with a joint injury involving heat and inflammation, it is best to have a medical professional diagnose it first. Once you have determined which muscles are involved and to what extent, you can teach the person to use Body Rolling to work the unaffected tendons of the inflamed muscles above or below the injured joint. Once the inflammation and swelling have subsided, the client can use Body Rolling to maintain the leg in healthy alignment.

The purpose of the following routines, then, is to restore full length and range of motion to all the leg muscles and to change the quality of bone that has become rigid due to excess impact. As direct pressure from the ball stimulates bone and increases circulation, the bone will soften, begin to breathe, become more permeable, accept nutrition, and become separable from other bones with which it articulates.

Leg Routines

For these routines, use whatever size ball is comfortable for you. It is important that you do all three routines (or four, if you include the iliotibial tract) on one leg first. When you finish working with that leg, compare it to the other, feeling the differences in both lying and walking and looking in the mirror to see the effects on your torso. After comparing visually and by sensation, do the same routines on the other leg.

Since there is less body weight on the ball when you work the posterior and anterior calf muscles, you may not feel you are affecting them; but if you wait and breathe long enough, you will feel them start to give.

The routines that follow are extremely detailed. However, you will find that when working with clients it is not necessary to be as muscle-specific with leg problems as it is for some of the other conditions discussed in this part of the book. The routines for the hamstrings and posterior calf muscles given below can be combined into one general back-of-the-leg routine; similarly, the quadriceps and anterior calf muscles routines can be combined into one front-of-the-leg routine. Most leg problems will be resolved simply by teaching people these two routines plus the routine for the adductors.

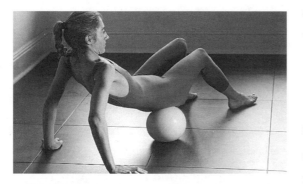

FIGURE 10.2

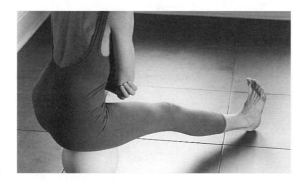

FIGURE 10.3

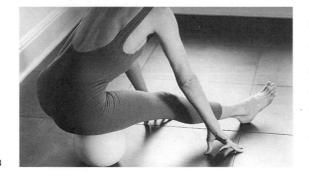

FIGURE 10.1

HAMSTRINGS ROUTINE

Start with the ball as high on your right hip as possible. With all your weight on the ball, roll down the gluteus maximus from all its origin points, in turn, toward its insertion at the gluteal tuberosity of the femur and the iliotibial tract (figure 10.1). Roll to and then along the ischium, stimulating the origins of the semitendinosus, semimembranosus, and biceps femoris muscles.

Slowly roll off the ischium, keeping some weight still on the bone but with the ball partly below it (figure 10.2). Wait and breathe, stimulating the release of the three tendons. Hamstring movement should start right at the origin points, so visualize these tendons softening and becoming more elastic. Slowly roll one-third of the way down the posterior femur (figure 10.3). Depending on how intensely you feel the stretch, bring your body weight and hands as far forward as you can to put as much pressure as possible into the hamstrings.

Since the hamstrings are formed by a group of three muscles, as you work down your thigh begin with the ball in the center, then roll both medially and laterally at each point. This helps separate the three hamstrings from each other, balancing the knee. Frequently an imbalance between the hamstrings makes the leg tighter on one side. Usually the biceps femoris is tighter, keeping the other two hamstrings from functioning fully and weakening the medial side of the knee.

Roll down to the knee slowly, in order to deeply affect the muscles. About halfway down you will feel a thickening at the linea aspera; this is the second head of the biceps femoris (figure 10.4). Wait at this point; applying pressure here will further release the lateral side of the knee.

For yoga students, working through the hamstrings this way is a great help in understanding the dynamics of the forward bend. As the hamstrings release the femur downward, you will feel a stretch in your lower back and in the deep lateral rotators. Two-thirds of the way down the femur, press the ball into the tendons of the two medial hamstrings.

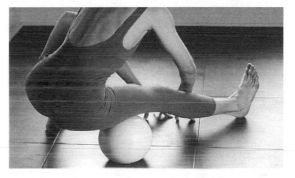

FIGURE 10.4

Roll down to the medial tibial condyle (figure 10.5). Here you are stimulating the insertions of the semimembranosus at the posterior medial tibial condyle and the semitendinosus at the

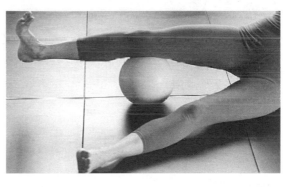

FIGURE 10.5

anterior proximal tibial shaft. Wait, feeling these muscles take their full length. You can flex and point your foot for additional release.

Now roll to the lateral side of the knee, releasing the insertion of the biceps femoris at the head of the fibula (figure 10.6). You might need to turn your leg outward to put more weight on this insertion. Again, wait and breathe.

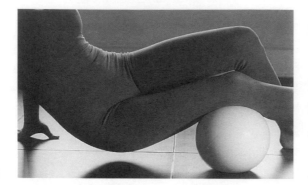

FIGURE 10.6

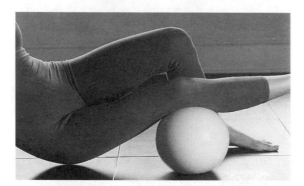

FIGURE 10.7

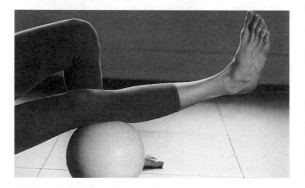

FIGURE 10.8

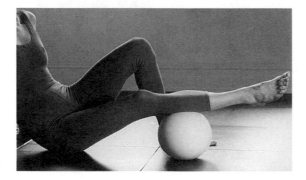

FIGURE 10.9

POSTERIOR CALF MUSCLES ROUTINE

Roll into the middle of the back of the knee and wait again, releasing intra-articular pressure. Visualize the ball sinking into the posterior knee, with the femur and tibia separating. Now roll laterally, to the lateral epicondyle of the femur (figure 10.7). This is the origin of the plantaris and popliteus muscles and of the lateral head of the gastrocnemius. Wait here to let their tendons release. Shortness in the biceps femoris will contract these muscles, which in turn will exert a powerful hold that turns the knee outward, restricting range of motion and weakening the medial side of the joint. Such a knee is vulnerable to injury.

Next, roll down from the lateral epicondyle of the femur to the head of the fibula. Breathe and wait for release. To release the origins of the soleus muscle, move the ball to the posterior head and upper shaft of the fibula (figure 10.8) and wait. Then roll posteriorly two-thirds of the way down the soleal line of the tibia and the interosseous membrane, placing the ball between the fibula and tibia (figure 10.9), and wait again.

To release the tibialis posterior muscle, roll back up to the head of the fibula, then posteriorly down the fibula again about one inch. Sink the ball deeply between the tibia and fibula at the interosseous membrane. To affect the muscle here you really need to visualize that the ball is sinking in between the bones. Roll down the tibialis posterior about two inches, then shift the ball slightly medially to put more weight on the tibia (figure 10.10). Here you are stimulating the flexor digitorum longus muscle, whose origin is on the posterior tibia. Now shift laterally to put more weight on the fibula (figure 10.11), stimulating the flexor hallucis longus muscle at its origin on the posterior fibula.

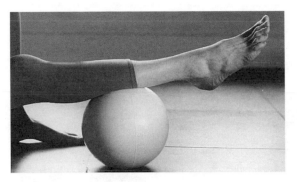

FIGURE 10.10

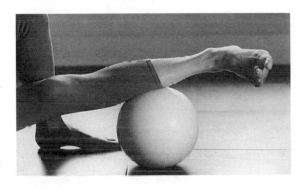

FIGURE 10.11

These three deep posterior calf muscles all have tendons that wrap around the medial malleolus and insert in the plantar foot. If these muscles do not have their full range of motion, foot flexion and range of motion will be restricted.

Roll all the way down to the calcaneus (figure 10.12) and wait, flexing the foot to increase the stretch. To work the peroneus longus and brevis muscles, roll the ball to the head of the fibula and then down into its lateral shaft, into the origin of the peroneus longus (figure 10.13). Roll down this muscle. About one-third of the way down, the ball will be affecting the origin of the peroneus brevis. Continue

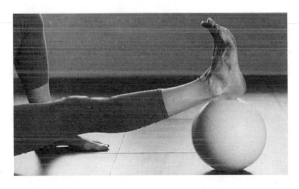

FIGURE 10.12

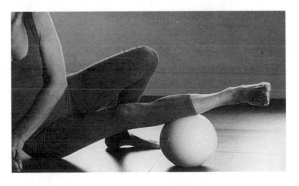

FIGURE 10.13

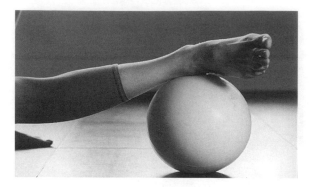

FIGURE 10.14

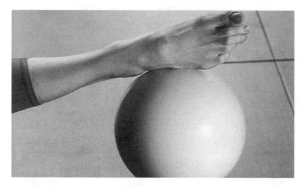

FIGURE 10.15

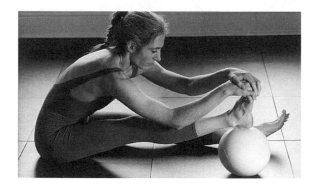

FIGURE 10.16

rolling to the lateral malleolus (figure 10.14) and wait. Then roll to the insertion of the peroneus brevis at the base of the fifth metatarsal (figure 10.15), and wait again.

Take the ball back up to the medial epicondyle of the femur and put pressure on the medial head of the gastrocnemius. Slowly roll down this muscle all the way to the calcaneus. As the ball rests on the calcaneus, the entire chain of muscles you have just worked is stimulated. For an increased stretch of the posterior calf, bend forward as far as you can to increase the release of all the muscles at the back of the leg (figure 10.16).

● QUADRICEPS ROUTINE

This routine will show you which individual muscles of the quadriceps group may be contracted or attached to the femur, pulling the other muscles toward it and restricting the movement of the whole group. I include the sartorius with the quadriceps group because you work it from the same anterior position.

The sartorius is the key muscle for knee alignment. If it lacks length and tone, the other muscles of the leg will be unable to take their full length. To release the origin of the sartorius, place the ball at the right anterior superior iliac spine (figure 10.17). Extend the leg; you should be able to feel a tug at the insertion of this muscle at the medial shaft of the tibia. Roll down the muscle, following its fibers toward the insertion at the medial side of the tibia (figure 10.18). Your intention is to free the sartorius from any attachments to other quadriceps muscles.

To release the rectus femoris muscle at its origin, place the ball at the anterior inferior iliac spine (figure 10.19). If you stretch the right leg out on the floor, you can feel the rectus femoris elongating all the way to its insertion at the patella and the tibial tuberosity. Because this is the most superficial muscle of the group, the deeper quadriceps all tend to become attached to it and move with its movement.

Now place the ball at the highest point of the anterior femur. To work the vastus lateralis, shift your body to the left so that the ball rolls laterally on the femur (figure 10.20). Support yourself on your right elbow and left hand, so that all your weight is directly on the origin of the muscle at the linea aspera on the posterior femur. Wait there, then roll down the muscle. At each point roll slightly anteriorly, then slightly posteriorly. This movement frees the muscle from the iliotibial tract, rectus femoris, and vastus intermedius.

Continue rolling in this manner about two-thirds of the way down the femur. Then bring the ball back up, place it on

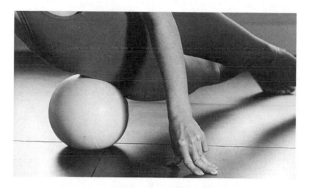

FIGURE 10.17

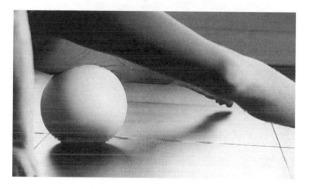

FIGURE 10.18

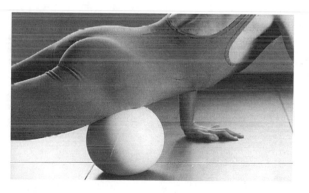

FIGURE 10.19

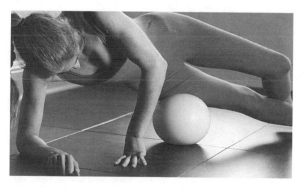

FIGURE 10.20

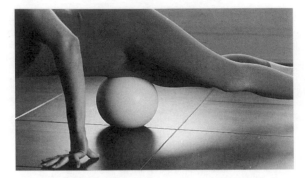

FIGURE 10.21

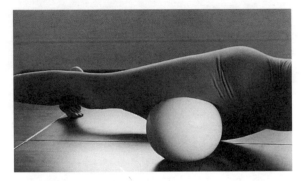

FIGURE 10.22

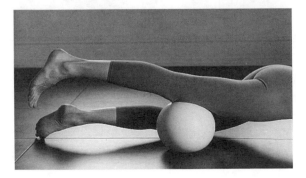

FIGURE 10.23

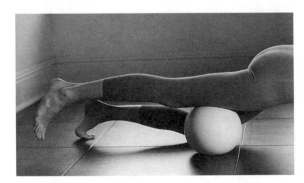

FIGURE 10.24

the origin of the vastus intermedius at the anterior lateral femoral shaft (figure 10.21), and let it sink in below the rectus femoris. To release the vastus intermedius, you need to visualize the ball sinking down to the bone. Maintaining this depth, slowly roll down the muscle with the same anterior-posterior movements that you used with the vastus lateralis. This time you are freeing the vastus intermedius from the vastus lateralis, rectus femoris, and vastus medialis. Roll two-thirds of the way down the femur.

Now place the ball at the origin of the vastus medialis at the linea aspera on the posterior femur (figure 10.22). Roll two-thirds of the way down the femur, again rolling posteriorly and anteriorly at each point. You are freeing this muscle from the vastus intermedius, rectus femoris, and adductors.

After releasing these muscles, place the ball about three inches above the patella, at the beginning of the common tendon of the quadriceps group (figure 10.23). Wait and breathe at this point so that the tendon can begin to release. This point may be painful—you will find that these muscles become more tightly attached to each other and to the femur as you approach the knee.

Roll to just above the knee so that

the ball is pushing the patella gently downward (figure 10.24). Wait here, turning the knee medially and laterally. The patella may be pulled upward by short quadriceps; this is a wonderful, safe way to bring it down to its optimal position.

ANTERIOR CALF MUSCLES ROUTINE

Without putting direct pressure on the patella, roll the ball down to the tibial tuberosity (figure 10.25). The weight of your leg on the ball should be directed into the tibia.

Wait and breathe, holding the intention of pushing the tibia down out of the joint to create more intra-articular space. With the ball directly on the bone, you can feel the release going on inside the joint. This is a direct bone effect—no muscle is involved.

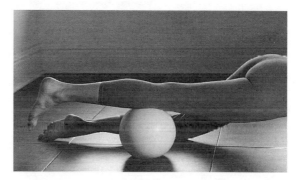

FIGURE 10.25

Now turn the leg medially so that the ball presses into the tibia and fibula (figure 10.26). Put greater pressure on the lateral shaft of the tibia and the interosseous membrane, the origins of the tibialis anterior muscle.

Move the ball to the origin of the extensor digitorum longus muscle at the lateral condyle of the tibia and the anterior shaft of the fibula (figure 10.27). Wait, allowing this muscle to begin releasing. Roll the ball down the muscle to the lateral malleolus, working to create space between the bones. You are simultaneously working the peroneus tertius muscle, which originates on the distal one-third of the fibula.

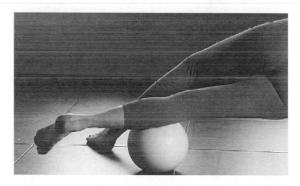

FIGURE 10.26

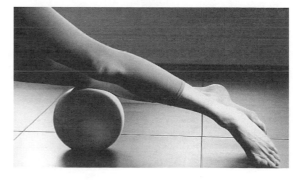

FIGURE 10.27

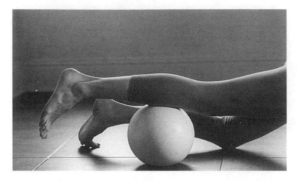

FIGURE 10.28

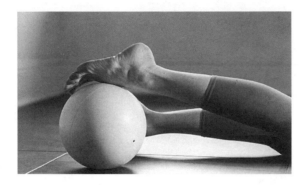

FIGURE 10.29

To work the extensor hallucis longus muscle, place the ball at the anterior shaft of the fibula, then roll down the muscle to the ankle.

Bring the ball back to the tibial tuberosity, again pushing it distally. With the weight of the ball on just the tibia, not on muscle, slowly roll all the way down the front of the tibia (figure 10.28). At the ankle, wait again. Then roll down, applying direct pressure first on the tarsal bones and then on the metatarsals (figure 10.29). Finally, roll out to the tips of the toes. With this movement you are releasing the insertions of the tibialis anterior, extensor hallucis longus, extensor digitorum longus, and peroneus tertius muscles. Wait and breathe, until you feel all the muscles in this chain releasing out to the toes. This is a subtle release, and you need a good thirty seconds to feel the tension in your toes letting go, the whole top of your foot warming up, and the muscles releasing up to the knee.

ADDUCTORS ROUTINE

Lying on your belly with your weight on your elbows, bend your right knee out from the

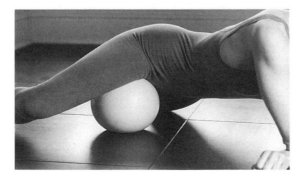

FIGURE 10.30

hip at a ninety-degree angle. Place the ball so that it presses into the pubis, pubic ramus, and inner thigh (figure 10.30), giving a general release to the entire adductor group.

Now place the ball at the anterior pubis on the origin of the pectineus muscle, the uppermost adductor (figure 10.31). Wait and breathe, sinking directly into this origin point. When you feel the tendon softening, put more pressure on the ball so that it sinks inward toward the muscle's insertion between the lesser trochanter and the linea aspera of the posterior femur. If the short, tight pectineus is contracted, it will cause contraction in the other adductors, preventing abduction of the leg.

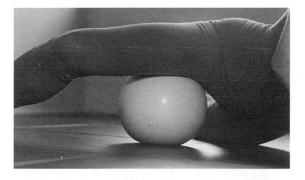

FIGURE 10.31

Next you will work the adductors longus and brevis and the gracilis simultaneously. Begin by rolling back to the anterior pubis, the origin of the adductors longus and brevis. Wait here, then roll out

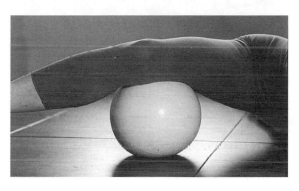

FIGURE 10.32

along the linea aspera of the posterior femur (figure 10.32), breathing and visualizing elongating these three muscles out to their insertions. The brevis inserts about one-third of the way down the femur; the longus inserts about halfway down. The gracilis also has its origin on the anterior pubis, and it inserts at the medial proximal tibia. Roll all the way down to this insertion.

To work the adductor magnus, which originates on the ischial tuberosity and the pubic ramus, place the ball on the pubic ramus and ischium. Keeping most of your weight on the ischium, roll down along the muscle's insertions between the linea aspera of the posterior femur and the adductor tubercle of the medial femur. This muscle, the largest and strongest of the adductors, often becomes attached to the semimembranosus and semitendinosus by connective tissue. Thus, when the semimembranosus and semitendinosus are restricted, they restrict the adductor magnus. Keep the ball at the adductor tubercle of the medial femur for twenty to thirty seconds, stimulating the entire adductor group.

ILIOTIBIAL TRACT ROUTINE

Place the ball at the anterior iliac crest, the origin of the tensor fasciae latae. Roll down to this muscle's insertion in the iliotibial tract (figure 10.33); now roll through the ili-

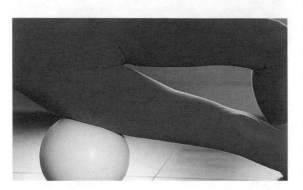

otibial tract to the knee. The iliotibial tract runs down the lateral thigh and inserts at the superolateral tibia and the head of the fibula. This routine tends to be painful, as the iliotibial tract is ligamentous and therefore less elastic than most other muscles. I do it less to release muscle than to stimulate the lateral side of the femur. I only include this routine

FIGURE 10.33

when I am leading clients through a release of the entire leg. Otherwise it is not strictly necessary, since a full release of the other three muscle groups is sufficient to stabilize the leg.

Working with Hip Replacements

Using Body Rolling following a hip replacement to keep all the muscles of the leg and hip as elongated and toned as possible will preserve range of motion in the hip and minimize excess pressure placed on the prosthesis.

When working with a client who has had a hip replacement, it is important to find out first which type of procedure was used. Different procedures sever different muscle groups. You must also talk to the surgeon to learn what type of prosthesis was used, what its mechanical possibilities are, and whether any screws might be protruding into muscle fiber.

Each year, as the procedure is improved, prostheses have a greater range of motion, but you still need to ask specifically what movements a given hip cannot make. Depending on what movements the physician advises against, warn your clients which positions are *not* recommended as they work the different muscle groups.

As in all types of surgery, after muscle is cut the surrounding tissues will contract toward the incision. In the leg, all the muscle groups will tend to adhere to the femur. The adductors are often left either completely atrophied because the lateral muscles are holding tightly, or they are completely contracted, pulling the femur toward the inner groin. The ball work can reinitiate function in all these muscles and free those attached to the femur.

Wait two months after the stitches are removed to begin the ball work. Start with a soft 8- to 10-inch ball, and use the leg routines given in this chapter. However, do not put any pressure or weight on areas where screws protrude into muscle.

Rolling the Feet with a Small Ball

As I noted earlier, the feet are the first part of the body to lose their circulation and range of motion, so keeping them stimulated is essential. Yet, no matter what type of exercise or other activity they are involved in, people mostly just let their feet go along; rarely do they think about giving the feet direct exercise. The more the individual foot muscles are worked, however, the more fully connected they become to the movements of the leg during walking, and the more conscious people can become about how they walk.

All the muscles that originate on the tibia and fibula insert in the foot or ankle. These muscles initiate foot movement and are always linked to the muscles that have both origins and insertions within the foot. The following routine, which uses a small ball to work the soles of the feet, benefits both muscle groups in several ways.

Because some people's body weight and energy are habitually collapsed down into the feet, putting pressure directly into the calcaneus transmits pressure upward into the talus and then into the tibia and fibula, actually creating space between those bones and taking pressure out of the ankle. This routine lifts energy up and out of the foot through the leg, reversing the process of collapse, stimulating venous blood flow, and reducing swelling in the ankles. Second, the routine directly stimulates the insertions of the muscles that run down from the calf as well as those that have both origins and insertions in the foot. Finally, as you roll you also stimulate all the reflexology points on the sole.

Use a solid rubber ball about two and one-half inches in diameter. It should have some give yet not be so soft that your weight will squash it completely. Do not use a tennis ball or other hollow ball. This routine is best done standing.

Place the ball under the center of your heel and put all your weight on it, making sure your arch is lifted and the ankle is not collapsed (figure 10.34). Slowly contact every point you can on the heel, sinking your full body weight into each point. You are stimulating release of the insertions of the gastrocnemius and soleus muscles on the calcaneus—notice how the pressure on your heel affects your calf and knee.

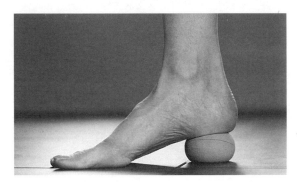

FIGURE 10.34

Roll off the center of the calcaneus into the tarsals (figure 10.35). The ball should still be pressing into the calcaneus while also sliding into the arch of the foot. As you roll off the body of the calcaneus you are releasing the origin of the quadratus plantar muscle, which inserts at the posterolateral border of the flexor digitorum longus tendon near the point where this tendon divides into four parts. If the quadratus plantar does not have its fullest possible movement, it will restrict the flexor digitorum longus and limit flexion of toes two through five. It is a key muscle in heel-arch separation.

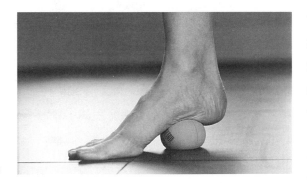

FIGURE 10.35

Shift your weight slightly laterally and wait. Here you are affecting the peroneus longus and brevis muscles. Now shift your weight medially to affect the tibialis posterior, flexor digitorum longus, and flexor hallucis longus muscles.

Maintaining the pressure on the medial side of the foot, push the ball up into the heel, then slide it off the heel and slowly work it toward the big toe, stimulating the flexor hallucis longus and the three muscles running down to the big toe: the flexor hallucis brevis, abductor hallucis, and adductor hallucis, which together keep the toe properly aligned. Put pressure on the proximal joint of the first phalange (figure 10.36), then roll out to the tip of the toe, pressing the toe down into the ball, separating it from the other four toes and forcing it to use these deep muscles.

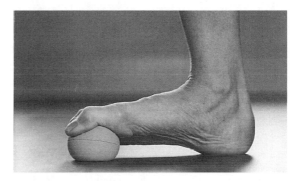

FIGURE 10.36

Now roll back to the point just off the heel but this time in line with the fifth toe. Roll down to the fifth toe, stimulating release of the abductor digiti minimi and the flexor digiti minimi brevis. Press the fifth toe into the ball. You are working the medial and lateral sides of the foot to get maximum width, which creates space for then working the middle toes. Most foot problems are due to narrowness through the foot that crowds all its structures together. This order of working will create more space for the middle three toes to spread into.

Roll back toward the same point on the heel, then slowly roll down the center of the foot, being sure to keep the ball in the center to stimulate the flexor digitorum longus. Roll to the toes and practice spreading them out around the ball and gripping the ball with them (figure 10.37). This action stimulates the lumbricals and interossei muscles, which are

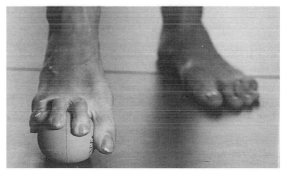

FIGURE 10.37

used to plantar flex the interphalangeal joints. In most people these muscles have lost their flexibility and thus greatly restrict toe movement.

This is a great routine to do when sitting for long periods, as on an airplane trip.

11

SCIATICA

The goal in treating sciatica is to take pressure off an inflamed, irritated nerve so that it can begin to heal. An injured nerve takes longer to heal than a muscle contraction or spasm, but some change in nerve sensation can be noticed right away. For example, after one or two ball sessions, sciatic nerve pain that originally went all the way down to the foot might only reach the knee. After another session it might stop at the thigh, and after a fourth session it might remain concentrated in the hip until the nerve heals. Relieving the pain completely might take a week of daily sessions (no more than one a day, however, since you do not want to exacerbate an inflamed nerve).

People commonly associate any pain running down the leg with sciatic nerve problems and assume they have sciatica. However, sciatica follows certain specific nerve paths and should not be confused with conditons involving other nerve paths. Thus, when someone comes in self-diagnosed with sciatica, the first thing to do is to determine exactly where the person feels nerve involvement.

The fourth and fifth lumbar nerves and the sacral nerve combine to form the sciatic nerve. This nerve runs through the greater sciatic foramen and down the back of the thigh. In the lower one-third of the thigh the sciatic nerve divides into the common peroneal and tibial nerves. The tibial division innervates the long head of the biceps femoris, the semitendinosus and semimembranosus, and the posterior portion of the adductor magnus, running down the back side of the leg and the plantar side of the foot to the tips of all five toes. The peroneal division, which innervates the short head of the biceps femoris, runs down the anterolateral calf to the first phalange of all five toes.

Nerve inflammation is caused by muscle compression that, over time, presses into nerve tissue and irritates it. In treating sciatica, therefore, you need to determine which muscles along the course of the sciatic nerve are in a chronically contracted state. To do this, ask your client to describe precisely where the pain is located. Pain due to sciatic nerve irritation can radiate to the lower back, the buttock, down the posterior or lateral thigh, and into the lateral posterior calf, ankle, and toes. If the pain is located someplace else, your client does not have sciatica and you must consider what muscles might be pressing on another nerve and need to be released.

There are two major causes of sciatic nerve irritation or inflammation. One is compression in the lumbar spine, which can irritate a nerve root. The other is severe contraction of pelvis and/or thigh muscles.

The following routine should relieve sciatica due to muscle contraction. If the client does this routine once a day for three days and feels no improvement or change, it indicates that the problem originates in the lumbar spine. In that case do the basic back routine up both sides of the spine (see chapter 5), focusing on creating as much length in the quadratus lumborum and latissimus dorsi and as much intervertebral space as possible. If the back routine provides no relief, the client should consult a physician.

Routine for Sciatica

Working on the side where you experience the pain, release the gluteus maximus at its origin along the sacroiliac joint and the superior gluteal line of the ilium, rolling the muscle fibers toward their insertion at the gluteal tuberosity of the femur and the iliotibial tract. Next, turn on your side and lean slightly toward the back to affect the gluteus medius and minimus, angling the ball slightly posteriorly on the highest part of the iliac crest (figure 11.1). Roll off the iliac crest into the origin of the gluteus medius on the external iliac fossa (figure 11.2). Wait, letting your weight sink into the ball.

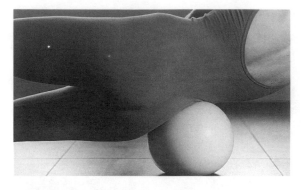

FIGURE 11.1

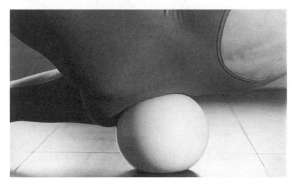

FIGURE 11.2

Then roll down the fibers of the muscle toward its insertion on the lateral aspect of the greater trochanter. Now roll back to the iliac crest and place the ball just anterior to the gluteus medius. Roll off the iliac crest, letting yourself sink deeper; you will feel a shorter, tighter muscle that will be a little painful. This is the gluteus minimus. Roll down to its insertion point at the anterior aspect of the greater trochanter. Stay there for a few moments.

Turn more onto your side and roll the ball back to the anterior superior iliac spine. You are now at the origin of the tensor fasciae latae. Roll down to its insertion in the iliotibial tract, then down the iliotibial tract about two-thirds of the way down the femur. At each point along the iliotibial tract, roll the ball slightly anterior, to separate the iliotibial tract from the vastus lateralis, and then slightly posterior, to the biceps femoris. This motion will prevent putting too much pressure on the iliotibial tract, which would be quite painful.

Now sit on the ball so that it presses into the ischium. Roll slightly forward so that you are pushing the ball superior to the ischium (figure 11.3), lifting the gluteus maximus to free it from the hamstrings. In many people the gluteus muscles drop due to

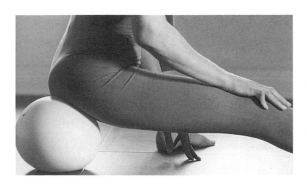

FIGURE 11.3

lack of use and become attached by connective tissue to the ischium at the point where the hamstrings begin. Lifting the gluteus maximus begins to separate the femur from the pelvis, taking pressure out of the pelvis and freeing the hamstrings to work separately, increasing range of motion of the femur.

Next, roll around on the ischium a bit to release the origins of the biceps femoris, semitendinosus, and semimembranosus muscles. Then slowly slide the ball down off the ischium into these tendons. Your hands are behind you taking some weight, your buttocks are sliding off the ball, and the weight of your torso is forward, to put more weight into the hamstrings (figure 11.4). The more you can lean forward, the more intense is this hamstring stretch.

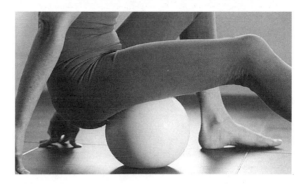

FIGURE 11.4

To release the semitendinosus and semimembranosus, roll toward their insertions at the anterior proximal tibial shaft and posterior medial tibial condyle, respectively. Bring the ball back up to the ischium and release the biceps femoris by rolling toward its insertion at the head of the fibula.

Roll back up again to the ischium and then along the pelvic bone to the acetabulum (figure 11.5), staying as close to the bone as you can and sinking your body weight against it. The pressure exerted into the ischium stimulates five of the six deep external rotators: the obturator internis and externus, gemellus superior and inferior, and quadratus femoris, all of which have their insertions at the greater trochanter of the femur. (The sixth lateral rotator, the piriformis, is stimulated when

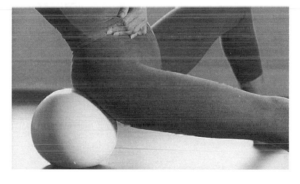

FIGURE 11.5

you release the gluteus maximus.) When you reach the acetabulum, wait and breathe, then take the ball away.

Finally, working the front connection, put the ball at the origin of the rectus abdominis at the pubic bone. Roll off the tendon into the abdomen. Staying close to the pelvic bone, roll into the anterior iliac crest (figure 11.6). Extend the leg out long on the floor, rotating the femur laterally and medially as you sink the ball deeper. Tell clients to imagine scooping the hip out with the ball. This stimulates the iliacus muscle.

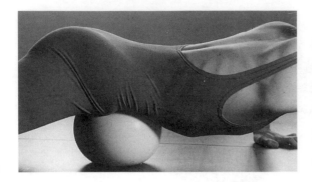

FIGURE 11.6

Often sciatica is due to a misalignment in the pelvis that puts more pressure on one side than the other. Thus it is important to do this routine on the other leg too, although you can work that side less intensively. Finish by rolling up the center of the spine.

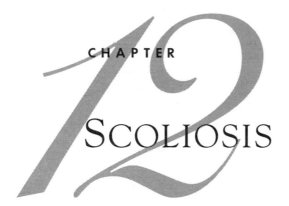

SCOLIOSIS

Scoliosis is an abnormal lateral curvature of the spine that occurs most frequently in the thoracic area, involving the ribs. Scoliotic patterns often have their inception during childbirth and are usually imprinted in the cranium.

In working with prepubescent girls with scoliotic dispositions I have found that many of their patterns developed due to a birth trauma that put pressure on the cranium. Usually the occiput and both temporal bones are rotated laterally in the same direction. This distortion in turn rotates the first three cervical vertebrae, transmitting the curve to the entire spine. The curvature will be in the opposite direction to that in which the head was pulled out during delivery.

For example, pulling the head out to the left places pressure on the right temporal bone so that this bone presses medially into the cranium, contracting the muscles on the right side of the cervical spine. As a result there is a twisting of the first few cervical vertebrae that rotates them to the left. This cervical curve will induce a scoliotic thoracic curve to the right. If such an injury is not noticed, the spine will continue to grow into the same torque it developed during delivery. During the preadolescent growth spurt and associated hormonal change, as the spine begins to grow more rapidly and solidify, a scoliotic pattern that has gone undetected becomes much more noticeable.

Most parents do not have the training to evaluate the alignment of an infant's head or the position of the eyes, shoulders, or pelvis. Even obstetricians and pediatricians generally are not trained to assess possible scoliotic misalignments in infants and children. To a concerned parent the physician's standard comment is, "She'll grow out of it." Consequently, many early signs of scoliosis are left untreated.

In working with scoliosis I first observe the location and degree of the curve, the point where it is most severe, and how it distorts the ribs, pelvis, or shoulders. Then I focus on creating length in the spine. I think of scoliosis as a distortion that prevents the spine from taking its maximum vertical space, and I consider my job to be giving the spine as much length as possible.

You can use the ball to relax the hold that the curve has on the spine, increasing mobility and decreasing any pain. The possible results will vary, depending on the degree of curvature. Ball work can soften some curvatures enough to give the person much more mobility and length in the spine and make the curve less obvious visually. In more severe cases, you can slightly soften the point of greatest curvature so that there is less discomfort and less restriction of movement, allowing the person to live more comfortably in his or her body. Finally, you can prevent the rigidity of the curve from increasing, and consequently stop the aging process that accompanies this progression.

I believe, too, that scoliosis usually has a powerful psychological effect. The torsion people with scoliosis must walk around with changes their focus, their presence, their whole perspective on life. The more rigid the curve becomes, the more difficulty they have in moving forward with ease in life. If they can keep that curvature as open and flexible as its nature allows, it does not have to limit their potential. And it is never too late to start.

Here again, the ball work is based on my premise that bone is malleable and movable. While it is true that, with scoliosis, the muscles hold tightly to the deviation in the spine, I believe that the real cause of the curve is the original distortion of bone, which is then reinforced by the erector spinae muscles adhering to the alterations. In general, any curvature anywhere on the spine will affect the entire spine as the other parts adapt to it. Therefore, in treating the condition you must treat the entire spine.

The general principle is to create length in both the lumbar and cervical spines and to visualize these two ends unwinding and creating space for the curvature to unwind into. You cannot begin where the curvature is—you must work first to create length at both ends to give the curve space to open into.

In treating scoliosis I work first with bone and then move on to tendon and muscle, rather than focusing initially on specific muscles. By sitting with the ball on each involved vertebra in turn, you create more intervertebral space and also release tight muscles.

Your client should start practicing this routine with a 10-inch ball. As the client grows comfortable working through the curves of the scoliosis and the curves begin to soften, she can switch to a smaller, denser ball, which will penetrate more deeply into the spaces between the ribs and into individual muscles.

You should explain to your client that a scoliotic pattern does not improve if left alone and that its severity will increase as the aging process increases general rigidity. People need to be educated about how to work with their own particular pattern of curvature. The routine described below takes about forty-five minutes, and should be done three times a week. It is appropriate for clients who are fully aware that, in order to achieve ongoing improvement, they must take on the responsibility of practicing it consistently.

General Routine for Scoliosis

Before doing the routine specific to the scoliosis, you need to begin with a general release of the entire spine and rib cage. The rib cage helps hold the scoliotic pattern in place; you will not be able to soften the curvature without loosening the ribs.

Begin by rolling up each side of the spine starting from the coccyx, as in the basic back routine (see chapter 5), keeping the ball as close to the spine as possible and really waiting at each point, working for as much sacral and lumbar length as possible. Think length: Visualize the spine softening and unwinding, with its length increasing from the lower back upward.

When you reach the point on either side where the curve is, begin working laterally. Press the ball toward the spine at each vertebra. Wait there, stimulating the release of the origins of the trapezius muscle at the spinous processes of the thoracic vertebrae, then sinking deeper to begin releasing the erector spinae muscles and loosening the articulation of each rib and vertebra. Breathe into this articulation.

Now angle the ball laterally, visualizing that you are ironing the ribs out flat. This will help to soften the scoliotic pattern. Breathe into the ribs and think about softening the bone and the quality of the curvature, forcing the breath into the point where the ball rests and into the intercostal muscles to create separation and movement in the ribs.

Next, roll up the sides. Begin on each side as in the basic side session (see chapter 6), but when you reach the ribs roll the ball posteriorly (figure 12.1) and breathe into the ribs, then roll the ball anteriorly (figure 12.2). Roll up one inch at a time, rolling to the back and then the front, waiting at each point, and breathing. If it is not possible to move in these very small increments, roll up one or two ribs at a time. As you breathe into the ribs in back and front, visualize the rib cage expanding and contracting like a bellows. Using your weight on the ball as a focus point, make sure you feel the ribs separate as you inhale and come together as you exhale.

Next, do the routine for freeing up the rib cage (see chapter 16) in order to loosen the ribs in front. At each point where the ball presses on the sternum you wait, then roll the ball onto the costal cartilage and wait, then roll the ball along the rib to push the rib outward (figure 12.3) and wait again. The costal cartilage is the source of the greatest elasticity in the rib cage; take advantage of this by visualizing the cartilage softening and

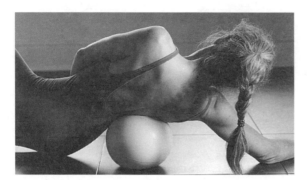

FIGURE 12.1

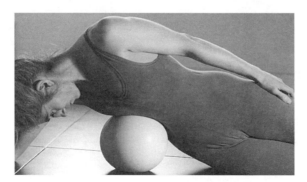

FIGURE 12.2

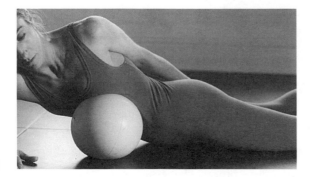

FIGURE 12.3

allowing the ribs to soften their curve. This in turn will allow the spine to release. The image is of trying to get the same bellows-like expansion here as in the side and back.

Now you are ready to work each side in detail to address the specific curvature. This time you will have the clear, focused intention of softening the ribs; you will hold longer at each point, breathing into the intercostal muscles to release them and create movement in the ribs that will help to soften the scoliotic pattern. Scoliosis is one case in which you use the ball differently on either side of the spine, depending on the type of curvature that exists.

THORACIC SCOLIOSIS

While all scoliotic patterns involve the thoracic spine, some occur lower down, resulting in a lumbothoracic curve, while others occur higher up and involve the cervical spine. A thoracic scoliosis involves curvature in the spine, sternum, and rib cage. In this case it is important to look at the alignment of the sternal attachments to the ribs and work the ball in the opposite direction from the curvature. (Because you can get greater release at the costal cartilage than at the attachments of the ribs to the vertebrae, I recommend beginning at the sternum.) For example, when the right side of the rib cage is twisted posteriorly and protrudes in back, the left side of the rib cage will protrude anteriorly toward the sternum. Accordingly, you would work the ball from the left side of the sternum upward and to the left, pushing the ribs out laterally.

Next you work on the back, with the ball pressing into the right side of the spine and then rolling out laterally toward the right side of the rib cage. Work up the entire thoracic spine from T12 to T1. Each "point" in this routine might be considered as every two or three ribs.

LUMBAR SCOLIOSIS

If the scoliosis has a pelvic involvement, you need to determine the angle of rotation of the pelvis and where and how the curvature affects the lumbar spine, sacrum, and pelvis. Begin by releasing the posterior pelvis, bringing length to the lumbar spine by working the pelvis downward. (For a detailed description of releasing this area, see chapter 8.) First release the origins of the gluteus maximus toward their insertions, visualizing that you are softening the entire sacroiliac joint on that side, working to straighten out the pelvis. Try to sense whether the sacroiliac joint is out of alignment. I tell people they can do this by noticing on which side they feel more tension in the gluteus maximus. They should then wait and breathe longer on that side.

Next, work the anterior side of the pelvis, elongating the rectus abdominis upward and then sinking the ball into the origin of the iliacus muscle on the inner surface of the ilium (figure 12.4). (For details on working these muscles, see chapter 9.) Stay

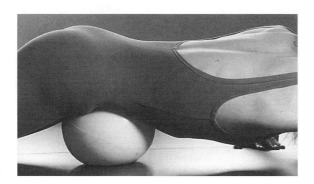

FIGURE 12.4

there for several breaths, feeling that you are twisting the pelvis back to center. You will also be working the external and internal oblique and the transverse abdominis muscles, which will be tightly contracted on the side of the curvature. As you work the anterior pelvis, you will be able to feel how the distortion of the rib cage may be affecting specific abdominal muscles and which of these muscles particularly contributes to holding the curvature.

Once the pelvis has been released somewhat toward its optimal alignment, the position of the legs in the hip joints will also need to shift. Now you must work the muscle groups of the legs to break their old holding pattern and allow them to adapt to the new position of the pelvis, otherwise they will not permit the pelvis to hold its new alignment. Although certain muscles will be more contracted, bringing the femur into alignment so that it can support the change in the pelvis requires working all the leg muscles and the six deep lateral rotators—use the routines in chapters 10 and 11.

Once the pelvis and legs are released, you can begin spinal work up each side of the spine, trying to create as much space between the sacrum and the lumbar spine as possible. Work the latissimus dorsi, quadratus lumborum, and posterior inferior serratus muscles in detail, according to the instructions in chapter 5. On the side with the greatest contraction, wait and breathe longer at the origin points of these muscles before rolling out toward their insertions.

When you reach the thoracic vertebrae, follow the instructions in the section on thoracic scoliosis above, working according to the curvature.

THORACOCERVICAL SCOLIOSIS

If the curvature is greatest in the first five thoracic vertebrae, the scoliotic pattern will affect the alignment of the cervical spine, shoulders, and head. In severe cases it can restrict shoulder movement, greatly restrict range of motion of the head and neck, and cause headaches, nerve impingement, and cervical herniation.

To treat this type of scoliosis, first evaluate shoulder and head alignment and range of motion at the shoulder. The distortion of the ribs will be greatest at the most extreme point of curvature. Usually the first four ribs are pulled upward, causing shoulder elevation and restricted movement. The ribs need to be worked downward to release the shoulder.

Begin by working up from the coccyx on both sides of the spine. Work the side opposite from the curve according to the basic back routine (see chapter 5). When you reach the thoracic area on the side where the curve is, begin rolling out laterally for three or four inches along each rib. Once the ball is level with the inferior angle of the scapula, roll laterally at each point to the vertebral border of the scapula. To release the infraspinatus and subscapularis muscles, roll over the vertebral border onto the scapula and out to the insertions of these muscles on the humerus (figure 12.5). (For a detailed description of this procedure, see chapter 14.)

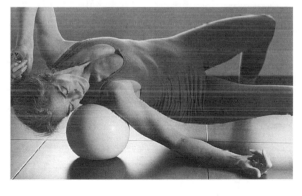

FIGURE 12.5

After releasing these two muscles, roll back to the spine and continue rolling up the origins of the trapezius to the occiput. Roll up the occiput to the sagittal suture, keeping the ball on the same side as the curvature. Wait and breathe here, working the shoulder on that side down away from the head. Slowly roll back down the occiput and

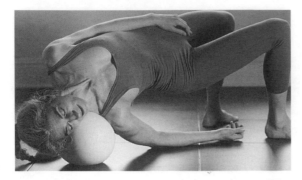

FIGURE 12.6

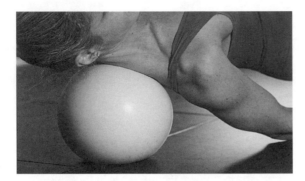

FIGURE 12.7

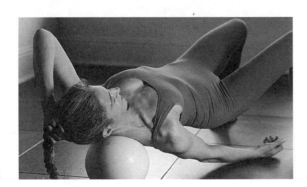

FIGURE 12.8

down the cervical origin points of the trapezius. Raising the hips, roll out toward the insertions of the trapezius at the acromion and the lateral clavicle (figure 12.6).

As you roll down the origins of the trapezius at the cervical spine, you are also stimulating the origins of the levator scapula at the transverse processes of C1–C4. From C4, roll out along the line of these muscle fibers to their insertion at the vertebral border of the scapula (figure 12.7), from the superior angle to the root of the spine of the scapula.

Next, release the rhomboids from their origins at the spinous processes of C7 and T1–5 to their insertions on the vertebral border of the scapula. Roll over these muscles several times, holding the image of spreading the scapula laterally and downward. Then go back to the origins and wait, sinking the ball into the spine to reach the deeper serratus posterior superior muscle, with origins at the spinous processes of C7 through T2 (figure 12.8). Raise the hips off the ground to exert maximum pressure on this muscle, visualizing the ball sinking all the way in to the underlying rib, exerting a downward pressure on ribs two through five and releasing the muscle toward its insertions at the lateral borders of these ribs.

The serratus posterior superior is a very deep muscle that has a lock on the four upper ribs; releasing these ribs downward creates tremendous freedom in the neck, shoulders, and back, and opens up the chest. So the intention here is to push these four ribs down, away from the cervical spine. The more movement you create in these ribs, the more freedom you give the shoulder joint. Unless you release these ribs, you will not be able to release the hold that the curvature has on the upper thoracic spine. All three serratus muscles are important for freeing the rib cage, but the serratus posterior superior has the strongest lock of all on the upper thorax.

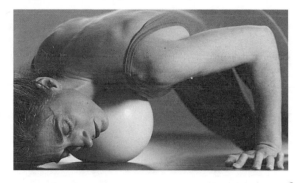

FIGURE 12.9

Since the shoulders and ribs are involved in a thoracocervical scoliosis, you should also do the basic side routine on both sides (see chapter 6).

The last part of the routine is to work on the anterior thorax. Do the basic front routine to elongate the abdominal muscles (see chapter 7), then move the ball up to the sternum and do the routine described for the sternum in the earlier section on thoracic scoliosis (see page 133). The shoulder will be elevated on the side of the scoliotic curve. To release the shoulder from the front, roll the ball

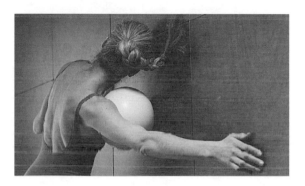

FIGURE 12.10

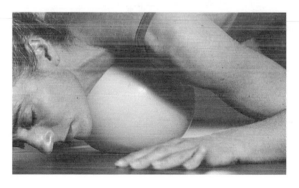

FIGURE 12.11

out laterally from the sternum until you reach the clavicle (figure 12.9). Raise your hips to exert maximum pressure on the clavicle and roll out along the clavicle to the shoulder with the arm extended along the floor (figure 12.10). Roll back along the clavicle to its attachment at the sternum (figure 12.11); then roll down the sternum along the costal cartilage to the level of the eighth rib. The arm on the working side should now be down along your side, with the other hand helping to support you.

Bring the ball back superior to the clavicle at a point one inch lateral to the

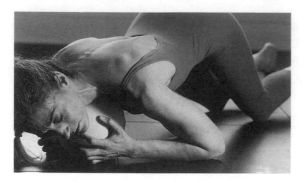

FIGURE 12.12

sternoclavicular articulation (figure 12.12). Push the ball down against the clavicle, roll over the clavicle with your weight pressing the ball into the first three ribs, then roll exerting a downward pressure on the rib cage as far as the fifth rib. Breathe into each point, pushing the ribs into the ball as you inhale and letting the ball sink into the ribs as you exhale, breaking their upward holding pattern. Continue to roll downward from point to point along the clavicle until you reach the shoulder joint. Keep your head turned to the opposite side.

CHAPTER 13

HERNIATED DISK

The intervertebral disks, composed of spongy cartilaginous material, make the spine flexible by providing intervertebral space. Years of weight-bearing and pressure lead to a slow degeneration of the disk, which gradually begins to bulge out of its natural space. A disk is said to be "protruding" when its annulus extrudes; it is said to be "herniated" when its nucleus protrudes. Herniation is more dangerous than protrusion, since there is likely to be more nerve involvement. Nevertheless, a protruding disk can cause as much pain as a herniated one.

The Body Rolling treatment for herniated and protruding disks derives from my basic philosophy of giving every part of the body its rightful space. Working with the ball to create space from vertebra to vertebra takes pressure off the disks, making Body Rolling an effective tool both for preventing herniated disks and for self-maintenance after a disk has been medically treated.

When dealing with lower back pain, it is essential to take preventive measures rather than waiting for the client's next flare-up. Lower back problems will not go away unless they are addressed. Often chronic lower back pain that goes untreated will develop into a herniated disk. People with chronic lower back pain might go for a year without a recurrence, and then suddenly find one day that they cannot even get out of bed and wind up being diagnosed with a herniated disk. Yet, by doing as little as twenty minutes of ball work three times a week, people can prevent major back problems.

In order to determine whether your client can use Body Rolling for a herniated disk, it is essential to see an MRI diagnosis so that you know exactly where the herniation is located. *If the disk material is pressing into the spinal cord, the disk should not be treated using the ball.* Once such a herniation has been cured by some other modality, however, the client can use the ball for self-maintenance work.

The key in treating a herniated disk is to use traction to elongate the area. As the spine lengthens, the disk is given space to move back into its rightful position. Physicians have used this principle of treating herniated disks through the use of traction for years. However, because they work by placing general traction on the whole spine, it can take many treatments to produce a lasting effect. By contrast, Body Rolling creates intervertebral space by restoring the functional memory of the erector spinae muscles, elongating and toning them from one vertebra to the next all the way up the spine, so the muscles can then support the intervertebral spaces.

This chapter addresses herniated lumbar and cervical disks. Thoracic herniations are rare, except when there has been a strong blow or an accident or in the case of a severe thoracic scoliosis. Most lumbar herniations are caused by wear and tear, while cervical herniations are usually due to whiplash injuries or other trauma, as well as to wear and tear. For both types of herniations I use the basic routine for working up the sides of the spine as described in chapter 5, except that in the area of the herniation I shift the weight slightly to the right when working the right side and slightly to the left when working the left side. In this way the ball maintains pressure on the transverse process of the vertebra above the herniation. Throughout, I work with the image of creating enough intervertebral space to allow the herniated disk to slip back into its proper place.

The routine described here for working with a herniated disk can be just as effectively applied to a protruding disk. Most people with herniated disks are in so much pain that they are willing to follow these intensive routines. My clients do them religiously every day for half an hour. For people who still have mild symptoms after surgery, as well as for those who have chronic symptoms of herniation, these routines offer tremendous alleviation of pain—the more people do them, the more relief they achieve.

Most lumbar herniations are the result of years of pressure exerted on the lower spine, the area of the back that takes the most abuse. Not only do gravity, weight, and bad posture take their toll, but we tend to rely more on the lower back than on the rest of the spine for strength in doing such activities as lifting heavy objects. Eventually the lower back simply gives out.

In response to a lumbar herniation, the sacrum usually becomes very rigid as it attempts to hold up the whole spine. In order to create intervertebral space in the lumbar spine, however, the sacrum must be able to drop downward, freeing itself from L5. To release a herniated lumbar disk, therefore, you must work upward from L5, lifting and separating each vertebra. To open up the sacrum, it is absolutely essential to start working at the tip of the coccyx and to roll up and down the sacrum several times.

The spine is a single entity. If severe compression in one area causes a herniated disk, the whole spine will be compressed to some degree. If one link goes, the entire spine is affected; a herniated disk creates a major weakness as the other vertebrae strain to do their job. Consequently, if a herniated lumbar disk goes untreated, or if it is treated surgically and intervertebral space is not created after the surgery, within five to ten years a second herniation is likely to appear, either just above the original disk or at the other end of the spine. By the same token, a client who has had surgery for a herniated cervical disk is likely to develop severe lower back pain within two to five years, and usually winds up with a herniated lumbar disk.

The pathological process is as follows. Just as with any surgical intervention, following laminectomy and diskectomy the tissue contracts during healing toward the site of the trauma. At the same time, that link loses its flexibility. Because this contraction and loss of movement create tension at that point of the spine, the vertebrae just above and below it are likely to begin having problems as well.

Whatever a person experiences at one end of the spine will also be experienced at the other end. Since a herniation results in a lack of space in the entire spine, you cannot simply treat it at one point; you must restore length throughout.

Because most of the spinal muscles move upward, as they do the following routines people should visualize releasing muscles at each vertebra and working to create length from the base of the spine all the way up by waiting, breathing, and pushing each vertebra upward. People who use this image achieve much more length through the spine than those who don't use it.

Routine for Lumbar Herniation

Use an eight- to ten-inch ball, medium-hard and not slippery. If after one month of practice your client wants to do more detailed work, he can switch to a smaller, denser ball. (This type of ball would be too painful to use initially.)

Begin with the basic routine of working up each side of the spine (see chapter 5), rolling up each side of the sacrum two or three times and noting any experience of discomfort or referred pain on either side. Roll up into the space between the sacrum and L5 and stay there. Most herniated disks occur here, between L5 and S1 or L4 and L5.

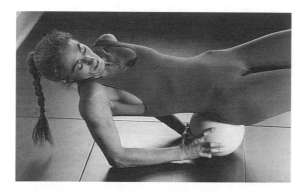

FIGURE 13.1

Before you continue rolling, lift your pubic bone slightly and use your weight to push the sacrum downward (figure 13.1). Breathe here, trying to visualize the separation between the sacrum and the lumbar spine. Take hold of the ball with both hands so you can control it. Roll it outward to spread the hip (figure 13.2), as in finding the quadratus lumborum in the basic back routine (see chapter 5). When you have rolled the ball as far laterally on the posterior iliac crest as possible, stay at that point and breathe. Then push your feet into the ground and use your hands to push the ball into the space between the sacrum and L5 (figure 13.3). This pushes the sacrum downward. At the same time, tilt your body to that side so you can apply lateral pressure to the spine, pressing into the spinous and transverse processes.

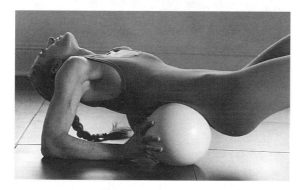

FIGURE 13.2

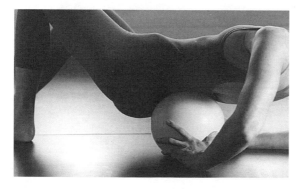

FIGURE 13.3

As you roll up to the next vertebra, again tilt your body toward the side, pushing the ball toward the spine with your hand. Using your hand to push while your body weight bears down to the side and into the ball is essential in this routine.

Once you are past the area of the involved disk, you do not have to use your hand anymore. Continue rolling up the spine, however, visualizing pushing the ball up into each vertebra, feeling the one below dropping down, then breathing into the intervertebral space. Roll all the way up to the occiput in this manner. As in the basic routine, focus on flattening out the lumbar and thoracic spines as you lay the vertebrae down on the floor.

Repeat on the other side. When there is a herniated disk there will probably be a displacement of the vertebra above or below. There might be lateral rotation or posterior or anterior slippage. So as you begin to roll up the second side, try to feel whether there is an area in the spine where a vertebra is displaced.

To help people perceive this you can explain that, when a vertebra is displaced, they will feel more sensitivity at that point. There will also be more resistance to letting go because the muscles are gripping, straining to hold the vertebra in its displaced position. Suggest that your client change the angle of the ball to put direct pressure on the displaced vertebra, trying to push it back into alignment, visualizing that she is creating space for it to slip back into place. To ensure that people maintain adequate space for the new alignment to hold, have them apply upward pressure on the two vertebrae superior to the displaced one, staying and breathing at each vertebra for twenty to thirty seconds, visualizing that they are taking pressure off the vertebra below that they have just realigned.

I also treat lumbar herniations by working the abdomen. When someone has a herniated disk that protrudes anteriorly or a displaced vertebra that has slipped anteriorly, this is often the best way to treat it. Sometimes there is so much external heat and inflammation that rolling up the back is too painful. In such a case I work solely from the front for a while.

To work the abdomen do the basic abdominal routine, starting at the pubic bone (see chapter 9). Rest here, feeling how pressure on the pubic bone begins to relax the sacrum. Slide off the pubic bone and immediately begin breathing, sinking the ball into the abdomen. Your image is of sinking in as deeply as you can, all the way to the anterior part of the lumbar spine. You will not actually get that far, but applying pressure to the front of the body in this way begins to relax the psoas muscles, which in turn will relax the lumbar spine. The longer you lie here, the more pressure you take out of your lower back and the more length you provide on the anterior side of the spine, creating additional intervertebral space.

Roll up to the navel. Stretch your legs and arms out as long as possible, visualizing that your back is completely flat as you lie on top of the ball; the ball is pushing your lower back out, getting rid of lumbar stress and any exaggerated lumbar curve. You are now stimulating the entire psoas major muscle. Visualize that its elongation is releasing the lumbar spine to its maximum length. Use your inhalations as well to expand the lumbar spine.

Remove the ball, roll over on your back, take a couple of deep breaths, and feel how differently your lower back lies on the floor. Is it flatter? Do you feel less discomfort?

Routine for Cervical Herniation

For working on the neck, use a six- to eight-inch, moderately hard ball.

Do the same intensive work on the right side of the sacrum and the lumbar spine as described above, then continue upward. Make sure you support your head with one or both hands as you roll up the thoracic area (figure 13.4)—this traction is essential in preventing any further irritation or pressure in the cervical spine. Your goal is to accumulate as much space as possible in the rest of the spine so that you can achieve maximum space in the cervical area, which is the hardest part of the spine to give space to.

Because the cervical vertebrae are smaller than those of the lumbar and thoracic areas, as you roll from the thoracic into the cervical area you will lose the sense of being able to feel each separate vertebra. At this point you are simply try-

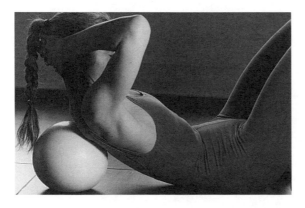

FIGURE 13.4

ing to create as much length as possible in the cervical spine as a whole. Roll through the cervical spine rather quickly, bringing the ball to the highest point of the occiput at the sagittal suture (figure 13.5). Pushing up on the occiput helps loosen its articulation with the first two cervical vertebrae. Stay at this point for one minute or so, working your shoulders down away from your neck.

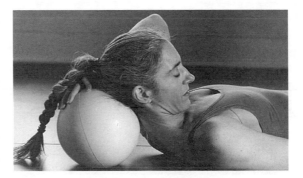

FIGURE 13.5

Now begin to roll the ball down the occiput toward the cervical spine. Lift your hips off the ground so that more of your body weight pushes against the ball. Keep your hips up as you roll off the occiput into the occipital groove, then laterally along the occipital ridge toward the mastoid process on that side (figure 13.6). Lower your hips and wait and breathe here. Now raise your hips again and roll medially toward the highest cervical vertebra that you can put pressure on with the ball, crossing the insertions of the splenius capitus at the mastoid process and occiput (figure 13.7). As you roll in

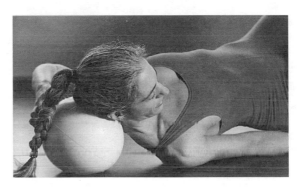

FIGURE 13.6

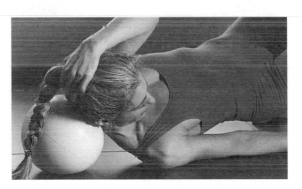

FIGURE 13.7

toward C1–C3, you are stimulating the release of the splenius cervicis at its insertion. Using the left hand, increase the traction at your head, bringing your chin in toward your chest. Maximum traction creates additional intervertebral space in the cervical spine. This traction is what allows you to apply pressure on the cervical vertebrae without further irritating or inflaming the herniated disk.

Begin to roll down from one transverse process to the next, tilting your head to the right so the ball exerts pressure on that side of the cervical spine (figure 13.8). You will

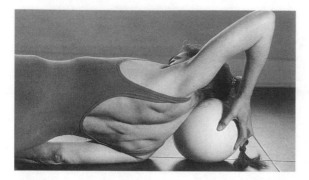

FIGURE 13.8

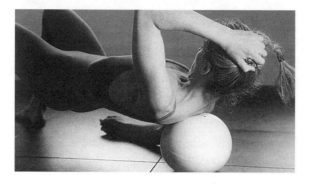

FIGURE 13.9

not be able to feel each vertebra individually at first, so visualize the ball pressing into each transverse process in turn; wait and breathe for twenty to thirty seconds at each point. To avoid getting tired, bring your hips down to the floor as you breathe at each point, then lift them as you move the ball again. Use one hand to hold the ball snugly against the side of the cervical spine, angling it into the transverse processes.

Continue rolling downward in this way until you reach the thoracic area. Then, as you roll down the thoracic spine, make sure you support your head with your hands, applying upward traction (figure 13.9). Roll to T5 or T6, then remove the ball. Rest, relax, and feel the differences between this side and the other.

Repeat the same routine on the left side.

Note that if there is a great deal of heat or inflammation, you should not roll directly through the cervical spine. Roll up to T1, then move the ball to the occipital groove and roll up from there to the sagittal suture. This will begin to create additional length in the cervical spine, reducing the heat and inflammation so that you will soon be able to do the more detailed work.

11

Shoulder
Problems

My basic principle for treating shoulder problems applies to any joint: Give length to all the muscles that either originate or insert at the joint. As I explained in chapter 6, shoulder problems begin in the hip. To resolve them, therefore, you must elongate all the muscles of the torso that interdigitate up to the shoulder joint: the latissimus dorsi, trapezius, anterior serratus, rectus abdominis, external and internal obliques, and pectoralis major and minor. These muscles provide the stabilizing forces from front and back that give length to the torso and position the skeletal structures of the shoulder joint in optimal alignment. Once these muscles are released, you can more easily access the specific muscles of the shoulder girdle in order to release them completely. In most cases this treatment will in itself largely resolve the problem. Any shoulder problem that persists must be dealt with more specifically.

The latissimus dorsi and trapezius muscles provide the length and width that help maintain correct posterior shoulder alignment. The longest and widest muscle of the back is the latissimus dorsi, which has its origins at the sacral and iliac crests, the thoracolumbar fascia, the spinous processes of T7–T12, and the posterior surfaces of the lower ribs, and inserts on the bicipital groove of the humerus. The trapezius muscle has origins on the spinous processes from T12 to T1 and from C7 to the nuchal ligament and the occiput. It inserts on the lateral one-third of the clavicle, the acromion process, and the scapular spine.

When the latissimus dorsi is contracted at its lower origin points, it pulls the shoulder downward, restricting shoulder movement. It also prevents release of the trapezius at that muscle's lowest origin points. This will cause excess tension in the upper one-third of the trapezius, resulting in restricted neck movement.

The latissimus dorsi and trapezius may both be contracted due to overuse, the contraction exerting a downward pull. This contraction creates a tight lock on the back, limiting general mobility and flexibility and also restricting range of motion within the shoulder.

In the front, the rectus abdominis, internal and external obliques, and transverse abdominis maintain length from the pelvis to the rib cage, keeping the rib cage lifted. Contracted or sluggish abdominal muscles pull the anterior thorax downward, restricting anterior shoulder mobility. Length in these muscles enables you to elongate the pectoralis major and minor, which are also essential for proper shoulder position.

The shoulder has the greatest range of motion of all the joints. It is a less stable joint than the hip, to which it is often compared. Whereas the femur's articulation with the pelvis is stabilized by the foot pressing into the ground, the arm is free-floating. Further, the hip joint is comprised of only two bones, the femoral head and the acetabulum, while the shoulder is comprised of three bones—the scapula, humerus, and clavicle—offering three possible articulations.

Because the free-floating arm moves with almost every action we take, it is difficult to stabilize the shoulder and easy to develop inflammation and joint irritation. The difficulty of stabilizing the shoulder is also one reason why it is harder to treat injuries in that area than in other joints.

Most shoulder injuries are due to years of repetition of a movement or movements that stress the joint. Tiny microfiber tendon tears brought on by the repetitive movement begin to develop. As time goes on the microtears weaken the muscle. Cartilage is worn away and synovial fluid production and circulation wanes. Eventually the person winds up in pain and is unable to move the shoulder. When a joint wears away, movement is limited to the range of the repetitive motion, and is sometimes decreased beyond even that.

Traumatic accidents cause other types of shoulder injuries. To treat these cases you need to analyze the direction of the blow and its impact on the alignment and the condition of the three bones of the shoulder joint, and determine which muscles are contracted or inflamed. Dislocations not caused by traumatic injury are usually the result of ligament problems and an extreme imbalance between certain shoulder muscles. In such cases the practitioner must determine which muscles are in extreme contraction and which are extremely low in tone, and then bring them back into balance as a functional unit.

In situations of trauma and dislocation from other causes, even if there is ligament damage, strengthening and balancing the muscles will stabilize the joint. Except when the ligament is actually torn, I have never seen a dislocated shoulder that could not be corrected by working through all the muscle groups connected to the shoulder girdle and rebalancing them.

It will be easier to correct shoulder problems and reeducate muscle in people who have good muscle tone, since muscle that is fit responds better to any type of treatment. Many women, for example, do not use their shoulder and arm muscles correctly; women often rely on their biceps, using their triceps minimally, if at all. The triceps consequently loses function and even begins to atrophy. Applying pressure with the ball to the origins of the triceps will be quite uncomfortable for such people, since these tendons have lost their memory of function. The process of treating shoulder injuries will be somewhat slower in these cases. In the following routines, people with less developed arm muscles will need to wait at each point much longer before their triceps understands that it can elongate and work.

The first routine described here elongates the muscles up the back, side, and front of the torso to give the torso its maximum length. The second two routines work with the shoulder girdle itself. A six-inch ball is best for working with the shoulder girdle; an eight- to ten-inch ball can be used in the torso routine.

Routine for Lengthening the Torso

This routine gives maximum length to all the muscles that keep the shoulder in optimal alignment. Each of the three parts will take twenty to thirty minutes.

UP THE BACK

When I give clients this routine, I emphasize that the latissimus dorsi is the key muscle for relieving shoulder problems. Since the latissimus dorsi runs from the lowest part of the spine all the way up to the arm, they will never get a full shoulder release if it is contracted. I demonstrate by asking them to raise the arm over the head the way they normally do. Most people only engage the upper one-third of the latissimus dorsi in this movement. I explain where the latissimus dorsi begins and ends, and tell them that it can elongate up from the pelvis, giving length to the whole back and raising the arm two to three inches higher than they have just raised it.

Then I ask them to raise the arm again while I place my hand on the lower part of the muscle to see whether they are accessing it or not. If they are not accessing it, I use my hands to lift the muscle up toward its insertion. I ask if they can visualize the muscle's full length and begin to elongate it all the way up the back themselves. This time the arm extends much more.

Begin with the basic back routine up the right side of the spine (see chapter 5). Roll up the sacrum, initiating release of the latissimus dorsi at the sacral and iliac crests, and then roll into the lumbar area, elongating the quadratus lumborum along the transverse processes of L5 to L1. As you roll up the quadratus lumborum, you will stimulate release of the serratus posterior inferior at its origins from L3 to T11, which in turn begins to release the trapezius at its origin at T12. Roll up the thoracic spine, releasing the entire length of the trapezius through to the occiput. Then roll to the sagittal suture at the top of the occiput. Wait here and breathe into the back of the neck, giving time for the muscles there to release.

Now roll down the occiput and down the right side of the cervical spine to T1 along the origin points of the upper trapezius. Lift your hips and roll out along the muscle fibers of the trapezius toward its upper insertion at the lateral clavicle and acromion (figure 14.1). Roll back toward

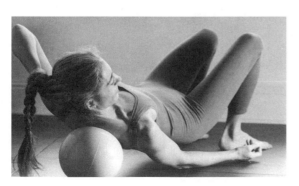

FIGURE 14.1

the spine and rest the ball between C7 and T1. Apply pressure by pressing the ball in toward the spinous processes of C7 and T1, the origin points of the rhomboid minor. Wait and breathe, then roll out toward the muscle's insertion at the root of the spine of the scapula, pushing out against the scapula.

Now roll back to the spine and press the ball into the spinous processes of T2–T5, the origins of the rhomboid major. (You can either work all four vertebrae at once, or press into T2 and T3, then go back and contact T4 and T5.) Supporting your head with your right hand, slowly roll down the rhomboid major to its insertion along the vertebral border of the scapula from the root of its spine to the inferior angle, pushing the entire scapula out laterally.

Next, roll over the vertebral border onto the scapula and to the origin of the infraspinatus at the infraspinatus fossa of the scapula. Stay at this point for about fifteen seconds with your body weight pressing into the origin, and breathe. Now roll through the infraspinatus muscle to its insertion at the greater tubercle of the humerus, and extend the arm outward, slightly above shoulder level (figure 14.2).

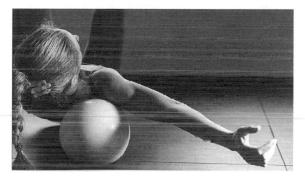

FIGURE 14.2

When you put direct pressure into the infraspinatus and roll out toward its insertion, you are also directly affecting the subscapularis muscle, which originates at the subscapular fossa of the scapula and inserts at the lesser tubercle of the humerus. In accordance with my theory that placing pressure anywhere on a bone releases all the muscles that have attachments on that bone, these muscles can be released together because they originate on opposite surfaces of the scapula and insert on opposite sides of the humerus.

Wait with the ball on the humerus for two or three breaths, then take it out from underneath you and relax, feeling the effects of the work you have just done. Then repeat this routine on the left side.

UP THE SIDE

Begin with the basic side routine (see chapter 6), rolling up from the right iliac crest, working to elongate the space between the iliac crest and the lower margin of the ribs. Here you are affecting the transverse abdominis muscle and the internal and external obliques. Slowly roll up into the ribs, avoiding the floating ribs. It is best to start with the ball placed between ribs eight and seven, where there is more stability. Try to stay directly on your side; wait for release, and breathe. Now roll slightly posterior, wait again, then slowly roll anteriorly. This begins to release the external and internal obliques at their attachments on the ribs.

Bring the ball back to the side and continue rolling upward, into the anterior serratus. This muscle originates from the upper nine ribs; at each of those ribs, muscle fibers move out to insert along the medial border of the scapula. You want to work the anterior serratus from each rib out toward its insertion on the scapula. Place the ball on the point on each rib where muscle begins, breathe, then slowly roll it back along the rib to the scapula, pushing the scapula posteriorly.

It is much harder to work the anterior serratus at the top three ribs, since there will be more tightness in the intercostal, latissimus dorsi, and pectoralis major and minor muscles, as well as in the muscles of the rotator cuff. The contraction of all these muscles produces a general tightening at the axilla. Go as high as you can into the axilla while feeling that you are still tracing the rib posteriorly. You have now worked the rib cage from front to back.

In describing the anterior serratus to clients, I explain that this muscle holds the ribs in balance and is also the most important muscle for increasing respiration into the side of the rib cage and creating maximum volume there. This muscle further determines the placement of the thoracic cage as a whole. When contracted it pulls the arm, shoulder, neck, and head forward. Therefore, work with an image of pulling the muscle upward from each of its origin points and backward toward its insertion at the medial border of the scapula. As you roll through the anterior serratus, even though you do not actually reach the medial border you push the scapula toward it, giving all the muscles that attach to the scapula more length and freeing the rib cage and central torso.

Next, roll the ball back down to rib nine, then roll slightly backward so that, though you are still lying on your side, you are pressing the ball at a side-back angle into the ribs (figure 14.3). This helps release the latissimus dorsi at its origins on the posterior surfaces of the lower ribs. Giving maximum length to the latissimus dorsi produces an immediate release of the teres major muscle at its origin.

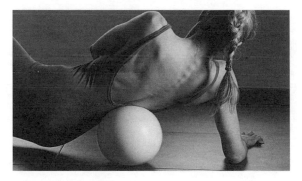

FIGURE 14.3

When you reach the inferior angle of the scapula, stay there a moment and breathe. Here you are stimulating the teres major, which originates on the posterior surface of the inferior angle of the scapula. This muscle acts almost as a con-

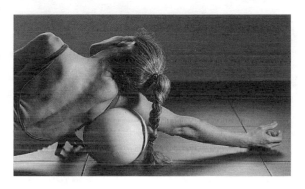

FIGURE 14.4

tinuation of the latissimus dorsi and has a similar action. When both of these muscles are contracted they pull the scapula downward, which in turn pulls the shoulder downward, restricting forward thrusting of the arm.

Finally, extend the arm to the side and roll up the lateral border of the scapula toward the insertions of the latissimus dorsi and teres major on the medial aspect of the bicipital groove (figure 14.4). Stay at the insertion point for several seconds, working to extend the arm further, then slowly release the ball. Repeat the routine on the left side.

UP THE FRONT

Begin with the ball at the pubic bone. Roll off the pubic bone and immediately angle the ball into the right side of the anterior pelvic cavity, tracing the inner side of the hip. Lengthen the right leg out as you roll up into the space between the anterior side of the iliac crest and the anterior side of the surface of the lower ribs, trying to extend your right leg and arm at the same time (figure 14.5). As you reach the surface of the lower ribs, sink the ball into the abdominal cavity. Here you are stimulating release of the diaphragm, the

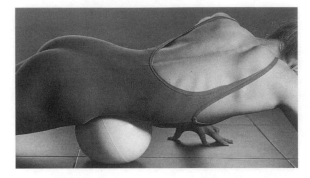

FIGURE 14.5

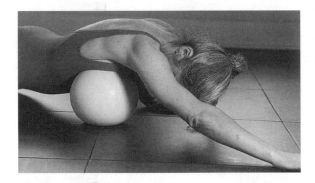

FIGURE 14.6

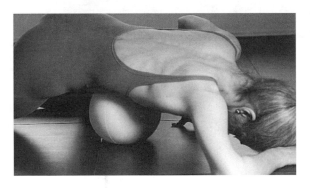

FIGURE 14.7

rectus abdominis, and the internal and external obliques. Angle the ball along the surface of the lower ribs toward the center as you lift the ribs upward.

When the ball reaches the xiphoid process, roll up onto the sternum, staying at its articulation with the costal cartilage on the right side. Here you are at the insertion points of the rectus abdominis at the costal cartilage of ribs five, six, and seven, and at the insertions of the internal obliques at the costal cartilage of the last four ribs. Stretch your right arm over your head and wait and breathe here, trying to initiate elasticity in the tendons of these muscles (figure 14.6). Then roll down slightly into the abdominal cavity to increase the release of these tendons (figure 14.7). This downward roll is important—it helps initiate a lift of the sternum, which is essential for keeping the thoracic cage upright and the shoulders aligned.

Roll back up onto the sternum and continue rolling up its right side over its articulation with each costal cartilage and about one-half inch outward onto each rib. At each point, shift your body so the ball presses first into the sternum, then moves out over the costal cartilage. Visualize the ribs expanding outward. Continue to roll up the sternum in this manner.

When the ball reaches the costal cartilage of the sixth rib, begin working the pectoralis major. This muscle has two heads. The sternocostal head originates on the sternum and the cartilages of the first through sixth ribs; the clavicular head originates on the medial half of the clavicle. Get up on your knees in order to apply more weight to the muscle. Begin at the origin of the pectoralis major on the sixth costal cartilage (figure 14.8), rolling it out to its insertion on the lateral aspect of the bicipital groove (figure 14.9). Repeat this action from rib six up to the first rib, beginning at the sternum and working out to the insertion point. On the last repetition, extend the arm out sideways and roll out the clavicular head of the muscle from the anterior medial clavicle toward the insertion at the bicipital groove (figure 14.10).

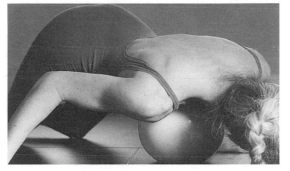

FIGURE 14.8

Roll back to the manubrium and move the ball up to the clavicular notch. Turn your head to the left side. Wait here, with the ball at the origin of the sternocleidomastoid muscle (figure 14.11), then lower your hips and slowly roll the ball with your hands up the sternocleidomastoid to the mastoid process (figure 14.12).

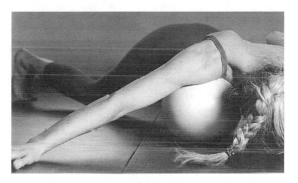

FIGURE 14.9

The pectoralis minor muscle is difficult to work with such specificity, especially for women, since it lies under breast tissue. However, extending the arm above the shoulder while working the costal cartilage of the third, fourth, and fifth ribs will also release the pectoralis minor at its origins.

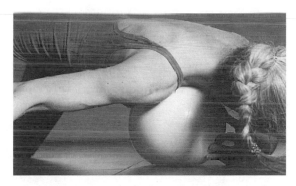

FIGURE 14.10

Slowly take the ball out from under you and relax on your back, feeling the difference between the right and left

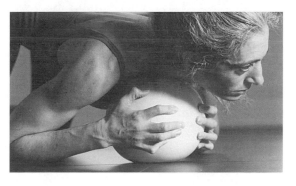

FIGURE 14.11

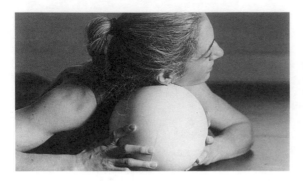

FIGURE 14.12

sides. Stand up and walk to feel the difference in the position of your shoulder, and assess whether your body feels more upright.

Repeat this series on the left side.

Routine for the Shoulder Girdle

This routine affects the muscles commonly referred to as the rotator cuff: the subscapularis, supraspinatus, infraspinatus, and teres minor. These are the muscles that guard the glenohumeral joint. This routine requires fifteen to twenty minutes for each side. Before doing this routine, clients should have already done the routine for lengthening the torso several times over the span of a couple of weeks in order to create sufficient length in the torso and to loosen up the shoulder.

Begin with the basic side routine up the right side (see chapter 6), paying attention to the specific muscles that give length to the torso: posteriorly, the quadratus lumborum, latissimus dorsi, and trapezius; anteriorly, the transverse abdominis and internal and external obliques. When you reach the rib cage, focus on freeing the anterior serratus; along with the latissimus dorsi and the pectoralis major, the anterior serratus is a key muscle that must be released in order to access the shoulder muscles.

Trace the anterior serratus as far up toward the first three ribs as you can. This helps widen the axilla. It is difficult to reach the first three ribs and quite painful to roll over them, so you might not want to go up that far to begin with; after doing this routine several times, you can challenge yourself to go farther.

Now roll down to the inferior angle of the scapula, with the ball pressing posteriorly (figure 14.13). Wait and breathe at the inferior angle, where the teres major has its origin. This muscle works with the latissimus dorsi and inserts next to it on the bicipital groove.

Roll up the lateral border of the scapula; you will be on your side but tilted backward (figure 14.14). Halfway up the lateral border is the origin of the teres minor; roll up this muscle to its insertion at the greater tubercle of the humerus. Now roll back down to the inferior angle of the scapula and onto the scapula, staying directly on top of it, your right arm extended over your head (figure 14.15). Here you are pressing into the infraspinatus muscle and also affecting the subscapularis below it. Wait and breathe. Then roll out to the insertions of the infraspinatus, supraspinatus, and teres minor at the greater tubercle of the humerus.

Roll back into the axilla (figure 14.16). This time you should be sinking deeper into the joint, affecting the insertion points of all the muscles of the rotator cuff and of the latissimus dorsi and teres major, as well as the origins of the coracobrachialis, biceps, and triceps. Now shift the ball anteriorly so that it presses into the pectoralis major, extending your arm as much as possible out on the floor (figure 14.17). Then move the ball posteriorly, pushing it into the lateral border of the scapula.

You have now created posterior and anterior space. Next you will create intra-articular space, focusing on separating the

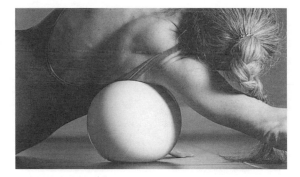

FIGURE 14.13

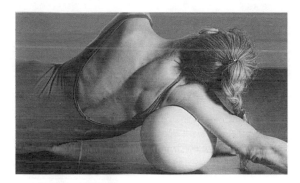

FIGURE 14.14

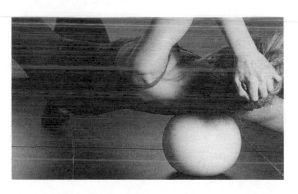

FIGURE 14.15

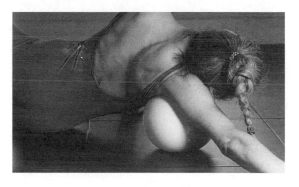

FIGURE 14.16

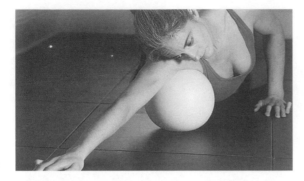

FIGURE 14.17

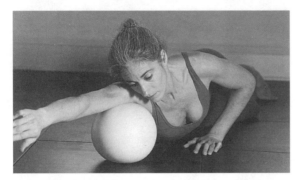

FIGURE 14.18

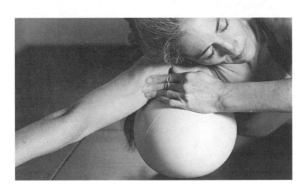

FIGURE 14.19

humerus, scapula, and clavicle.

With the ball in the center of the armpit, push it directly upward into the glenohumeral joint (figure 14.18). Putting this direct pressure on the humerus, scapula, and clavicle in this way will release all the tendons attached to all of these bones. To get even more specific releases, you can do detailed work on additional muscles that may be involved in shoulder problems: the coracobrachialis, biceps, triceps, and deltoid.

Coracobrachialis. When this muscle is contracted upward it pulls the humerus upward, restricting joint mobility; it also contracts the first three ribs upward, which in turn contracts the scalene muscles and tightens the neck. The coracobrachialis originates at the coracoid process and inserts on the medial surface in the middle of the humeral shaft.

To work this muscle, keep the ball in the axilla. You will not be able to reach its origin, but the pressure of the ball up into the joint begins releasing the origin nonetheless. With your left hand, press the medial surface of the humerus toward the muscle's insertion (figure 14.19).

Biceps. This commonly overused muscle can easily shorten, along with the coracobrachialis, and pull the humerus upward. Because it inserts on the radial tuberosity, it can also restrict range of motion of the elbow.

The biceps has two heads. The short one is shared with the coracobrachialis and can be released with that muscle. The long head begins at the supraglenoid tubercle; to release it, with the ball in the axilla squeeze the bulk of the biceps between your left thumb and fingers, stretching the muscle toward its insertion (figure 14.20).

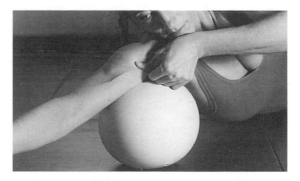

FIGURE 14.20

Triceps. This muscle has three heads. The long head originates on the infraglenoid tubercle of the scapula, the lateral head originates on the posterior humerus above the spiral groove, and the medial head originates on the posterior humerus below the spiral groove. To release the triceps, rotate your right arm with the ball in the axilla, so that the palm faces upward (figure 14.21). Press the ball into the scapula as close to the glenoid cavity as possible; you will be stimulating the long head. Reach your left hand over your right arm and grasp the body of the triceps from the back, rotating it upward while pulling it down toward your elbow (figure 14.22). Holding it in that position, roll the ball down your right arm an inch or two. This stimulates the lateral head. Roll down the posterior inferior humerus and rest the ball in the bulk of the muscle (figure 14.23). As you wait and sink deeper into this point, you will affect the medial head.

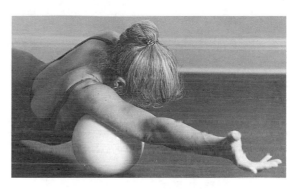

FIGURE 14.21

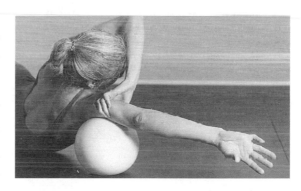

FIGURE 14.22

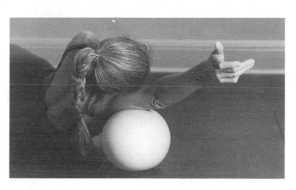

FIGURE 14.23

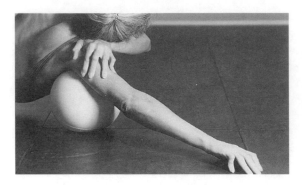

FIGURE 14.24

Deltoid. This muscle has origin points on the spine and acromion of the scapula and the lateral one-third of the clavicle. To stimulate these points, bring the ball back to the center of your armpit. Use your left hand to put direct pressure down on these origins, at the same time pressing toward the muscle's insertion at the elbow; rest the weight of your head on your left hand to increase the pressure (figure 14.24). Pressing down on the deltoid helps create intraarticular space, elongating the humerus out and down from the clavicle and scapula.

Take the ball away from the armpit. Lie on your back, rest and relax. Then get up and walk around, looking in the mirror to compare this shoulder with the other.

Repeat this routine on the left side. Even though only one shoulder may be injured, for the sake of maintaining balance the other side must also be worked. However, it is not necessary to work the uninjured side with the same degree of muscle specificity.

Finally, after doing such detailed work it is essential to end the session by rolling up the center of the spine.

Frozen Shoulder Routine

This routine gives people with a frozen shoulder who are in such pain that they are reluctant to move it a passive way to initiate movement and create some intra-articular space. The bones in the joint that are stuck together begin to separate, bringing increased fluid flow to the joint. This is a safe way to work toward joint mobility without increasing irritation or inflammation.

When working with clients with this condition, I explain that they have three bones that fit together to form the shoulder joint. When these bones are too tightly held together by short, contracted muscles, shoulder movement is restricted and bone may be rubbing on bone, causing inflammation and pain. I give them the image of the ball as a lever prying open the space between the three bones.

Hold a six-inch ball between your right elbow and side while stretching your head to the left (figure 14.25). This stretches the upper trapezius, supraspinatus, scalene, and sternocleidomastoid muscles. Breathe deeply into the right side, visualizing the ribs expanding, the intercostal muscles releasing, and the whole area becoming softer and more flexible. With the left hand, pull the right forearm to the

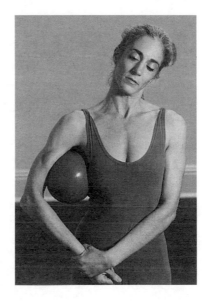

FIGURE 14.25

left so that the ball presses against the right side. Focus on pushing the ribs out into the ball on each inhalation, pressing the ball into the arm. This helps create space in the shoulder joint; it also releases the serratus anterior, intercostal, latissimus dorsi, trapezius, sternocleidomastoid, and scalene muscles, and stimulates a slight release of the biceps, triceps, and coracobrachialis muscles.

If you find this easy, move the ball closer to the armpit. Repeat the exercise until you can get the ball all the way up into the armpit, each time working strongly with the other arm to create traction in the joint. You can also try holding the ball more to the back and to the front. Visualize breathing into the shoulder, separating its three bones and allowing synovial fluid to lubricate the joint and restore its mobility.

15

NECK PROBLEMS

The first thing to look at when someone comes with a neck problem is alignment. When people complain about neck pains, they are usually referring to the back of the neck. However, as with every other aspect of the body, the key factor is balance. Because the neck is circular, we need to bring balance to its whole circumference. When you are evaluating why someone is hurting in a particular place, the question to ask is: "What other muscles do I need to bring into balance so these muscles aren't overworked and straining?"

To answer this, you need to find out how your client is using his body for the largest number of hours a day. Does he have a desk or telephone job, or sit at a computer? People with phone jobs tend to hold the phone only on one side. This pattern becomes so ingrained that even if they get headphones they still keep the head tilted to that side.

What's more, almost all of us hold our heads slightly forward. This position keeps the trapezius muscle in a continuous state of overuse, cutting off circulation into the head and altering the natural curve of the cervical spine. As you walk, your feet should be leading your body, but most people do everything "head first."

A properly aligned head is held so that the ears are directly in line with the shoulders and the chin is tilted slightly downward. In this position the cervical spine has its greatest length, and the muscles at the back of the neck are working in balance with those in front. Keeping the muscles of the neck as long as possible also activates the pectoralis muscles so they can perform their function of holding up the front of the rib cage. Once the pectoralis muscles are engaged, the shoulders open back and down, releasing tension from the trapezius. The opening of the chest also increases lung capacity and brings more circulation into the brain, enhancing mental clarity.

As an educator, your role is to make people aware of their patterns and give them possibilities for changing them. If you just work on them or even teach them to use the ball, there are still many hours each day when they can forget about their neck position. Once your clients have the feeling of a healthier alignment in the body, even though they will not be able to maintain it continuously at first, when they lose it they will take notice and be able to find it again.

In treating neck problems, the entire cervical spine needs to be elongated, not just the back of the neck. The muscles in the front of the neck can inhibit elongation of the cervical spine even more than those in the back. The powerful sternocleidomastoid muscles play the greatest role in maintaining proper neck alignment. If they are not given their maximum length, they will pull the neck and head forward. When you hold your head forward, as people do for almost any kind of task, you lose elasticity, shortening the muscles in the front of the neck. At the same time you overuse the muscles in the back, creating tightness and rigidity in the cervical spine.

Using the ball in the front of your neck gives you the sensation of how the muscles in that area function. When they are working properly, they take pressure off the back of the neck and also release the deeper muscles in the throat and anterior cervical spine. The ball is a great way to introduce people to a part of the body that most have no awareness of. Going into the front of the throat is often a psychological challenge. Many people have a fear of choking, gagging, being unable to breathe, or being strangled. The ball work shows them how such fears manifest physically in extremely tight muscles. They can then work on themselves to soften this area, helping release those deep fears.

The second element to determine in evaluating a neck complaint is the level of tension in the neck and its specific cause. Most neck problems are stress related, deriving from a person's most frequent activity, usually their work. The position in which someone holds his head while performing his work activities governs the specific muscular pattern of tension and, therefore, the nature of his neck problem.

If your general approach to a client's neck tension is not bringing about any noticeable change, get more information about his life, especially what other parts of the body might be involved in the stress on the neck. Daily tension built up over a long period of time usually goes to the neck. Some people have so much tension in their heads because of the nature of their mental processes and general way of being that the cranial tension causes all the muscles in the neck to contract. For others, neck tension is caused by physical exertion—some people keep the neck extra tight during exercise. Find out what a client's sport is and if possible observe his workout to see how he is using his neck during that activity.

High blood pressure implies added pressure in the chest, neck, and head. In addition, severe temporomandibular joint syndrome will prevent any work done on a client's neck from lasting if the syndrome itself is not addressed. Upper gastrointestinal tract stress or tension that begins with swallowing can cause deep internal spasms from the neck down into the stomach. Still another cause of neck tension is injury such as whiplash.

Treating Neck Problems

To avoid injury to veins or arteries, most massage schools teach students not to go deeply into the front of the neck. However, with Body Rolling you are never putting direct pressure onto any specific structure; you are giving length to the entire area, creating more space for the organs and muscles. This will actually promote greater circulation to the head.

Three routines for releasing neck tension follow. Because you cannot release the neck without releasing the spine, always begin a neck session by working from the base of the spine. The more release you can achieve in the lower spine, the greater the release will be once you roll up to the neck and head; you will not achieve as much release by simply putting the ball in the back of the neck. Rolling up both sides of the spine will also enable your clients to feel how the way they habitually position the head throughout the day affects each side differently.

Because it is one of the primary areas where they first notice tension, most people easily feel a release in the neck area. When they do the basic back routine they will immediately feel that the neck is more relaxed.

For these routines, work with a six-inch ball, which fits more easily into the neck.

BACK OF THE NECK ROUTINE

Do the basic back routine up one side (see chapter 5), rolling up through the occiput. Then slowly roll back down the occiput into the neck, angling the ball into the cervical spine. With your head tilted so that the ball presses in toward the spine (figure 15.1), wait and breathe, then slowly roll the ball laterally, using the occipital ridge as a guide, with the ball half on the occipital ridge and half below it. As you do this, you cross the splenius capitis and splenius cervicis muscles, as well as the trapezius and levator scapula. Roll the ball out toward the mastoid process (figure 15.2), and as you do so, begin turning onto your side. When the ball is over the mastoid process, wait and breathe—the sternocleidomastoid, splenius capitus, and longissimus capitus muscles all have attachments here.

From the mastoid process, slowly roll the ball down the side of the neck to the level of C3 (figure 15.3). Then roll back toward the spine until the ball is again pushing into the spine, approximately between C3 and C5. Roll down a bit

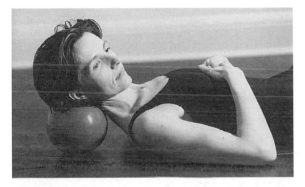

FIGURE 15.1

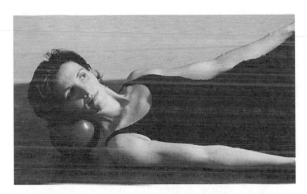

FIGURE 15.2

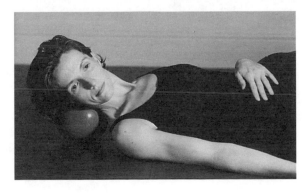

FIGURE 15.3

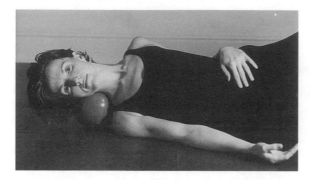

FIGURE 15.4

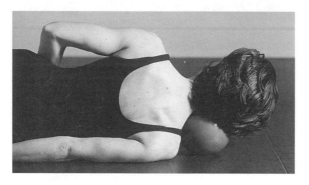

FIGURE 15.5

farther so the ball is at the lower cervical vertebrae and T1. Angle the ball in toward the spine, wait and breathe, then roll all the way around to your ear, turning your body so that when the ball reaches the line of the ear you are lying on your side with your lower arm in front (figure 15.4). Here you are releasing the upper one-third of the trapezius and the levator scapula. To get a more intense stretch in the neck, move the lower arm behind you (figure 15.5). Now you are releasing the pectoralis major, scalene, sternocleidomastoid, and deltoid muscles.

Initially it is difficult to sense each individual vertebra in the cervical spine, so as you angle the ball in toward the spine, visualize that you are affecting one specific vertebra and that the erector spinae muscles at that vertebra are subtly releasing. Then move down to what you sense is the location of the next vertebra.

Sometimes when there has been an injury to the cervical spine, one vertebra will feel larger or protrude more than the others. If you stay with the ball pressing into that vertebra and breathe, you can begin to break up the scar tissue around it and soften the restriction in that area.

Bring your arm in front again and roll slowly back around toward the spine. From T1 roll one more time straight up that side of the spine to the top of the occiput. This time the cervical spine will experience an even greater release.

Repeat this routine on the other side.

FRONT OF THE NECK ROUTINE

The critical repositioning for relieving neck tension is an upward movement of the sternum. To demonstrate this to yourself, stand up and press the fingers of both hands into the point right above the xiphoid process, pushing upward. Wait there for about thirty seconds. You will notice that your shoulders drop, the trapezius muscles relax back and down, the pectoralis major and minor lift and open toward their insertions in the shoulder, the sternocleidomastoid begins to release from its articulation at the sternum, the neck moves backward and elongates, and the chin drops.

Move your fingers up the sternum, maintaining the pressure. The neck continues to elongate and the holding patterns of the muscles in the back of the neck begin to release. This is the effect you intend to create in working up the sternum with the ball.

Place the ball just above the xiphoid process and roll up the center of the sternum to the attachments of the clavicles (figure 15.6). Wait and breathe at this point, where the sternocleidomastoid originates. Keep the pressure of the ball on this point for a good thirty seconds, then slowly try to sink the ball into the point just above the clavicle (figure 15.7), using your hands to keep the ball from sliding up into your neck. Your weight should be partly on the clavicle and partly just above it, not in the upper part of the throat. Wait and breathe here, focusing on releasing the back of the spine between T1 and C7. This is the point that corresponds to the point where the ball is on the front; there is often a restriction here. Feel this area begin to open.

Lift your head and push the ball in toward the clavicles, stretching the front of the neck out to its maximum (figure 15.8). Now lay the neck down over the

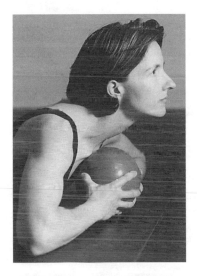

FIGURE 15.6

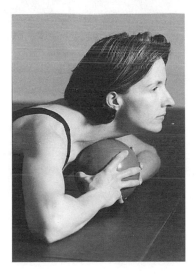

FIGURE 15.7

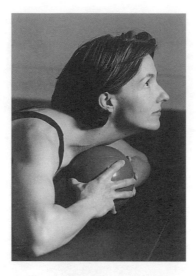

FIGURE 15.8

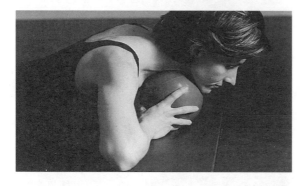

FIGURE 15.9

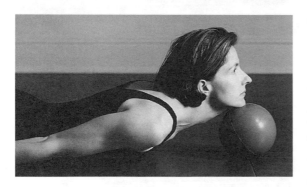

FIGURE 15.10

ball (figure 15.9), visualizing the front of the neck spreading outward and downward around the ball. Coughing is a normal reponse to sinking into the throat this way. Let go of the ball, unless you are feeling too much weight on the front of your neck. If that is the case, keep your hold on the ball, allowing your arms and elbows to take some of the weight.

Now bring the ball all the way to the tip of your chin (figure 15.10). For the greatest stretch of all the muscles at the front of the neck—including the scalenes and the platysma, the muscle responsible for the earliest wrinkles at the neck—keep your arms down at your sides, working your shoulders down away from your neck. Take several deep breaths into the front of the neck.

Next, move the ball a bit below the chin, and using your mandible as you did the occipital ridge in the previous routine, slowly trace the inferior aspect of the mandible with the ball out to the mastoid process (figure 15.11), rolling slightly onto your side to put more weight on the mastoid. Keep your lower arm down at your side, working the shoulder away from the head. Wait and breathe, applying pressure with the ball on the mastoid process. Here you are affecting the insertion of the sternocleidomastoid, stretching it away from the sternum. Finally, roll along that muscle back to the sternum (figure 15.12), supporting yourself with the other hand on the floor.

Do the same routine on the other side.

In giving this routine to your clients, you want them to feel how releasing tension in the front of the neck will relieve tightness in the back of the neck. You also want them to recognize just how much tension they might store in the front of the neck. Without giving too much technical detail, you can tell them that the sternocleidomastoid, which runs from the sternum to the mastoid, is important for proper head placement. Keeping it elongated and flexible will give fullness and length to the front of the neck and relieve much of their neck discomfort.

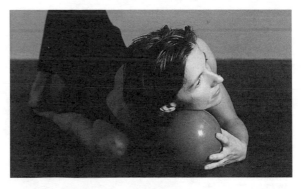

FIGURE 15.11

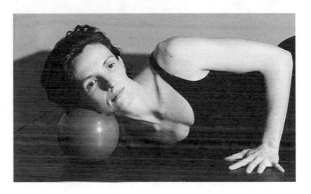

FIGURE 15.12

Emphasize that the direction of release is from the center of the neck out to the mastoid process. In order to be sure people stimulate the important attachments there, show them where the mastoid is. Since this is such a difficult area to work on, I tell people to visualize breathing into the whole front of the neck, feeling it soften, expand, and fill with light. By softening and opening this area they are creating a free flow of energy between the head and the rest of the body.

ROUND-THE-NECK ROUTINE

Doing this routine will tell you which muscles are involved in a neck problem and how the holding pattern has distorted them. Often people will notice that the side where they hold the phone all day will be short and the other side of the neck will feel strained, again demonstrating that the muscles affected by a pattern of tension are never just the ones where you feel the hurt.

This routine also helps people realize that, as a result of habitual patterns of work or other activities, the neck muscles tend to become fixed in one direction, making it difficult to turn the head in the opposite direction. To break this pattern, you need to roll around the entire neck in both directions.

This routine affects the deep as well as the superficial muscles of the neck. However, the muscles you can actually feel as you roll are the trapezius, the levator scapula, the splenius capitus and splenius cervicis, the scalenes, the sternocleidomastoid, and the platysma.

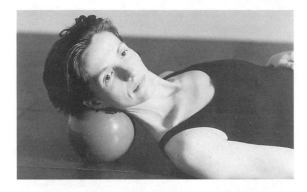

FIGURE 15.13

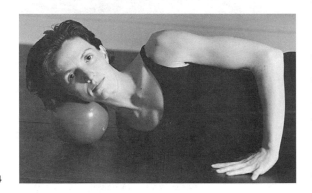

FIGURE 15.14

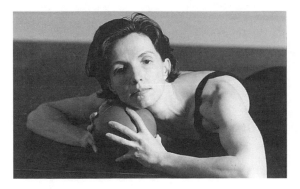

FIGURE 15.15

This routine begins with releasing both sides of the spine all the way up (see chapter 5). Then, with the ball on one side of the neck, angle the ball in toward the cervical spine. Make sure it is occupying as much of the length of the neck as possible. Slowly roll the ball out laterally and begin turning your body onto that side (figure 15.13). At first your arm is in front of your body and you are working your shoulder down away from your neck. As the ball approaches the line of the ear, begin bringing the arm behind you (figure 15.14). This affects the scalenes and the sternocleidomastoid. Roll slowly toward the center of the front of the neck, using the mandible and clavicle as guides, with the ball resting between them (figure 15.15). If you are feeling too much pressure, take some of the weight on your hands and elbows.

As you approach the center of the front of the neck, press the ball against the side of the larynx; this action affects the esophagus and trachea. These three structures, which should be separate from one another, tend to become stuck together and immovable. Visualize that you are separating the trachea, esophagus, and larynx and softening the connective tissue that usually binds them together. Wait here, breathing into the area and visualizing loosening up connective tissue so these structures can move freely.

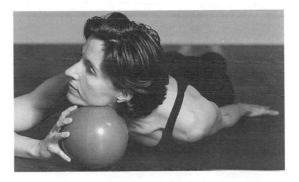

FIGURE 15.16

Let the ball roll over the center. Then, with the arm behind the body, slowly turn and roll across the other side of the throat (figure 15.16). Roll toward the mastoid process. As the ball goes behind the ear, bring your arm in front of you (figure 15.17).

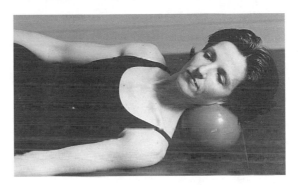

FIGURE 15.17

Turn over toward your back as you roll the ball toward the spine (figure 15.18). Continue until the ball is pushing into the other side of the cervical spine. Wait, and breathe.

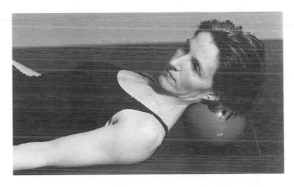

FIGURE 15.18

Finally, begin rolling around the neck again, this time in the opposite direction. Roll all the way around, finishing the routine by rolling the ball up the center of the back of the neck to the top of the occiput (figure 15.19). Holding the ball in place with one hand, raise the other arm overhead and wait there, breathing and focusing on your sensations.

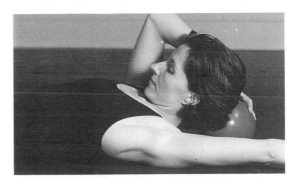

FIGURE 15.19

Now that you have done all this work on the cervical spine, it is in a release pattern. Holding it for a while with maximum traction will effect much more release.

Unless you experience your own holding pattern, it is difficult to understand what you need to do to release it. This routine provides an experiential self-awareness exercise. Once you have performed the round-the-neck roll in both directions several times, you will be aware of what your particular holding pattern is and which side—left or right— you need to work more intensively in order to dissolve it.

16

FREEING
THE
RIB CAGE

This chapter presents three routines that laterally expand the rib cage. Creating horizontal space is critical for freeing the hold of the ribs at the sternum and spine—this is what gives maximum vertical space to the thoracic and cervical vertebrae.

The rib cage is an area of the body where we naturally begin to harden against any type of threat; it bears some of our strongest armoring. The rib cage protects our heart, our lungs, part of the liver, and the upper gastrointestinal tract. Even more important, our emotional life is seated there. Blocked emotions may be carried in any part of the body, but nobody gets through life without the rib cage becoming armored. We all hold some kind of emotional scarring or psychological imprint there, resulting in a tightly contracted and rigid area that will eventually restrict movement in every body part that is connected to it—the head, neck, arms, and even the internal organs. The more contracted the rib cage is the more inhibited breathing becomes and the less oxygen and blood circulation the upper body receives.

The rib cage becomes restricted or even immovable quite early in life; its pattern tends to get fixed as early as age three. This pattern is often copied from the child's parents. When children are shouted at, hit, or pushed, the rib cage is the area they pro-tect by retracting the arms and shoulders.

When people want to know more about somebody, there is generally a particular part of the body that they look at. I look at the rib cage, for much of our identity is expressed there. The rib cage can reveal who a person really is—as when it is concave, with the shoulders and head dropped forward, telling you that this person is unsure of himself, unable to expand and take his space in the world. It can also tell you that someone is trying to project a persona unlike what she feels inside—as when the rib cage is thrust forward but has little breath in it and little movement, signaling that this person wants to create the impression of self-assurance and success.

In terms of function, the rib cage shapes itself according to the pattern in which we hold the body for the greatest number of hours each day. Even our breathing pat-tern adapts to the way our rib cage is held, often cutting off the flow of the breath into the upper ribs, shoulders, head, and neck. Therefore, in order to relieve pressure in a person's shoulders, head, and neck, in most cases you need to release the rib cage so that breathing can occur throughout its entire dimension. When beginning to work on a client's rib cage, it is important to first observe the rib cage during normal breathing to determine where it has limited or no movement.

Many problems in the body are connected to the rib cage. In the case of a person with asthma, for example, the chest is so tight that it has almost no elasticity. This is in part due to a spastic reaction to being unable to breathe; in the muscle pattern of that reaction the intercostal muscles, diaphragm, and lungs all contract. The routines in this chapter will help asthmatics free the hold the rib cage has on their breathing.

Many large-breasted women have no space between their breasts because they unconsciously contract the rib cage to hold the weight of the breasts. This is not a healthy pattern—the chest is locked, leading to restricted circulation and lack of func-tion in the internal musculature. The rib cage should be expansive and freely moving to support the breasts. Using these routines to open the thoracic cage makes the inter-costal muscles elastic, allowing the ribs to move and the sternum to expand to its nat-ural width. When you release the hold the costal cartilage has on the sternum, the ribs can expand laterally. Then the pectoralis muscles can hold up the front of the rib cage, including the breasts, as they are meant to do. This restoration of function will give the breasts more space and freedom.

Problems in the thoracic spine, such as a displaced vertebra or general vertebral compression, cannot be completely cured without freeing up the rib cage. Nor can you totally eliminate a shoulder problem if the ribs are held tight and high. One of the most difficult conditions for a body-therapy practitioner to treat is a frozen shoulder. While you can begin to release the muscles of the shoulder girdle, the locking of the upper rib cage will keep you from freeing these muscles completely and mobilizing the shoulder adequately. Constriction in the shoulder girdle must be approached by freeing up and repositioning the individual ribs, something most body-therapy practitioners are not trained to consider. From these routines you will learn that it is possible to move and soften bone—and change its position— just by putting direct pressure on the bone and having the intention of changing it.

There should optimally be a certain amount of space between each of the ribs. Check on yourself by using your finger to follow one rib from front to back as far as you can. Now check the next rib. In checking two or three ribs, you will likely notice a significant difference in the amount of space between them in different places. In fact, at some points you might feel no space or even notice ribs overlapping. When the rib cage can move freely, all the intercostal spaces can be more or less equal and the intercostal muscles can expand to their maximum during inhalation.

To accomplish all these changes, you must start by working on bone, not muscle.

Working on Bone

The rib cage is the first part of the body that becomes rigid in response to life experience. This rigidity develops early and persists, restricting most aspects of movement in everyday life. Emotions deeply embedded here will often make cartilage as rigid as bone, for when held in a contracted state over a long period, the costal cartilage becomes equally hard and inflexible. Once this happens, the intercostal muscles never develop their full capacity for expansion.

When the rib cage is frozen, more weight bears down into the pelvis, which can contribute to lower back problems. But when the ribs are free and flexible, the rib cage supports itself. There is a feeling of energy moving up and through the chest instead of being stuck inside the chest, with all the weight bearing downward. Freeing the rib cage allows the muscles of the torso to become toned and elongated, creating more space between the hips and the rib cage. However, since the thoracic cage is composed of more bone than muscle, in order to create this space you must first work on bone and cartilage, then work out into muscle.

The routines given here will increase breathing capacity and overall vitality, remove restrictions from the thoracic and cervical spine, and realign the head above the torso. You will be working to feel the sides of your rib cage expanding from the sternum laterally and from the spine laterally. You will also be freeing the ribs from the hold of the abdominal muscles and freeing the ribs and clavicle from the muscles of the neck and cervical spine. By restoring horizontal space to the chest this work increases the vertical flow of energy up the spine, which in turn increases the energy flow out into the shoulders, arms, and hands. Bringing more energy into the arms and hands provides us with more utilizable creative energy.

Because the ribs attach at both the sternum and the spine, thoracic spinal limitation must be treated from the front as well as from the back. The costal cartilage has enormous potential to become elastic, which means the size of the thoracic cage can be considerably enlarged. You can expect to see and feel literally the whole rib cage expand and contract with the breathing, just like a baby's. You are not fully aware of how a restricted rib cage limits your breathing and energy flow until you begin to notice change. Once you feel more freedom in the ribs, it is hard to imagine not having it.

Because the chest is so rigid, the first step in working on the rib cage is to soften the costal cartilage. I start at the inferior body of the sternum and work up the center line to stimulate the sternum to take its maximum size. This work also begins to change the quality of the bone. Then I work up each side of the sternum, along the line where the costal cartilage attaches to it, waiting and breathing at each point, imagining that the cartilage is expanding and stretching outward, opening up the ribs.

As you wait at these points, you also begin to feel the connection between the front and the back of the body. With the ball on the area of the sternum that corresponds to a spot in the spine that is difficult to work on, you might, for example, experience in the sternum exactly the same feeling of discomfort that occurs in that spot on the back. This usually happens when you keep the ball on the costal cartilage/rib attachment for a long time. As you wait and breathe, you can feel the attachment at the spine that corresponds to where you are on the costal cartilage. The reasoning mind jumps in to note the connection: By releasing the rib/sternum connection in the front, you can release the corresponding vertebra in the back. This experience is consistent with the theory that pressing anywhere on a bone will release its other points, even if you are not directly on the point of desired release.

For the following routines, use an 8- or 6-inch ball that is soft enough to rest on at each point. Usually you will feel what some people call "good" pain; the sensation may be one of tenderness or heat. The pain should not be excruciating. If it is, choose a softer ball or slightly deflate the one you are working with. Generally when people put pressure on the ribs with a ball, they know right away if that particular ball is too hard to use.

It is not necessary to do all of the following three routines in a single session. Since the rib cage has been more or less soldered into a certain position for years, it does not simply release like muscle; you will need to work on the rib cage a bit at a time. One day you can release the ribs from the spine and on another day focus on the sternum. As always, be sure to finish each session by rolling up the spine.

This is an advanced series of routines —those who choose to practice it should feel no pain or restriction in the lower back, should have achieved noticeable length in the torso, and should have done some work on the legs before they begin this work. At that point the body will need more horizontal thoracic space in order to further increase its length. As the body grows accustomed to the work, it becomes easier to do intensive, detailed work on the rib cage.

Back-of-the-Rib-Cage Routine

Begin by doing the basic back routine up the right side (chapter 5). When you reach the posterior inferior rib cage between T11 and T12, support your head with one hand

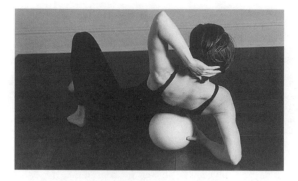

FIGURE 16.1

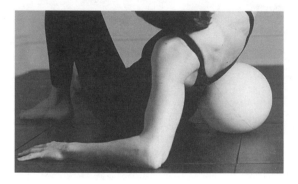

FIGURE 16.2

and press the ball in toward the spine, tilting your body to the right (figure 16.1). Let your weight push the ball between T11 and T12, visualizing space between the two vertebrae and the corresponding tubercles of ribs eleven and twelve. Breathe, expanding your rib cage out away from the spine. Now tilt toward the left and roll over the ball, applying pressure so that the ball pushes the ribs out to the right (figure 16.2). Roll out three inches from the spine. Continue supporting your head. Roll the ball back to the spine, then roll up one to two ribs and repeat this procedure until you reach the inferior angle of the scapula. Try to focus on one rib at a time. The ball will actually be touching two or three ribs at once, but focusing in this way will enable you to apply more weight on one of them and eventually to separate it from the ribs above and below. Because the ribs can be so tightly held together at first, you initially need to work them in groups.

From the point on the spine level with the inferior angle of the scapula, roll out laterally, opening your right arm out at about a forty-five-degree angle. Do not roll over the scapula itself, but visualize pushing it out away from the spine. Push the breath into the space where the ball is, focusing on sending the breath into the ribs under the scapula to expand them.

Now roll back in toward the spine, letting your weight press the ball into it. The thoracic vertebrae in the area between the scapulae are usually much tighter and have less mobility than those lower down. Since it is difficult to separate them, there will probably be only three points in this area where you will wait and breathe. (Try using a smaller ball if you want to get in deeper.) Because this space is so narrow—you will be rolling only an inch or two between the scapula and spine—it is important to wait longer at each point, again pushing the breath into the space where the ball is and expanding your rib cage laterally.

At the last point in this area, where you will affect the first three ribs, lift your hips off the ground and hold the ball with your left hand (figure 16.3). Angle the ball inward toward T1–T3, then roll out through the trapezius to that muscle's insertion at the acromion and spine of the scapula (figure 16.4). Due to the strong superior pull of the trapezius, levator scapula, rhomboid, and serratus posterior superior muscles, the first three ribs often become fixed in an elevated position. Your lifted hips direct your weight down-

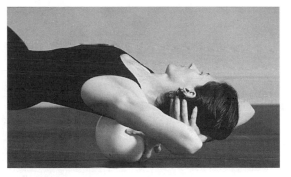

FIGURE 16.3

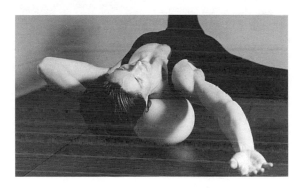

FIGURE 16.4

ward and out, pushing the upper three ribs down from the shoulder and neck. To exert sufficient force on these ribs, the hips must be fairly high.

Repeat the routine on the left side.

Front-of-the-Rib-Cage Routine

I introduce this routine to clients by telling them that, although they do not feel it, at the point where the ribs meet the sternum there is a more elastic material—the costal cartilage—that can give their ribs more freedom of movement, and this cartilage is what the routine will affect. Ribs one through seven, which insert from T1 through T7 posteriorly and attach anteriorly to the sternum, have less mobility because their costal cartilage is smaller. Ribs eight, nine, and ten have longer costal cartilages, which attach to the cartilage of rib seven rather than directly to the sternum, and attach in the back to T8–T10. Thus, the band of ribs below rib seven has greater possibility for expansion.

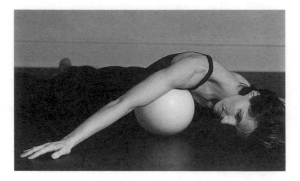

FIGURE 16.5

Place the ball at the center of the sternum, just above the xiphoid process. Wait and breathe, then move the ball exactly to the point where rib seven articulates at the costal cartilage with the right side of the sternum (figure 16.5). Tilt your body to the left so that you are almost falling off the ball and your weight is pushing out to the right, separating the ribs away from the sternum. Breathe here, visualizing the costal cartilage becoming more elastic. Your hips are flat on the ground, but your upper body is lying on its side.

Again, although you might well be touching two or three ribs at once, your intention is to affect the costal cartilage of each rib separately. Roll the ball outward along each rib. Women should roll it as far as they can without rolling over the breast; men can roll all the way to the side of the body. Use your right hand to keep the ball from sliding out from under you.

Roll along the length of one rib after another, from rib eight to the clavicle. At each point, first wait and breathe with the weight of the ball angling in toward the sternum, then roll laterally, pushing and breathing outward into the costal cartilage.

As you get closer to the clavicle the costal cartilage becomes much tighter, so you need to keep the ball at the sternum longer before rolling laterally. Remain at each point for twenty to thirty seconds. As women move the ball above rib five, they can roll out farther laterally because the ball is no longer touching breast tissue.

When you reach the origin points of the pectoralis major muscle at the costal car-

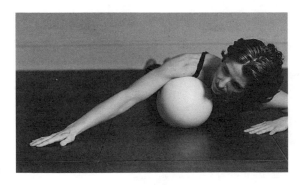

FIGURE 16.6

tilage of rib six, extend your right arm out to the side and roll from the costal cartilage toward the insertion of this muscle at the lateral lip of the bicipital groove of the humerus (figure 16.6). Bring the ball back to the fifth costal cartilage and roll along the muscle fibers toward the same insertion. Repeat this procedure on the next four ribs. Then roll down the humerus a few inches (figure 16.7), stretching the muscle to its maximum. This movement also initiates release of the origins of the biceps (both heads) and coracobrachialis muscles.

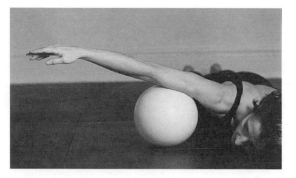

FIGURE 16.7

Bring the ball back to the manubrium. To put additional pressure on it, get up on your knees and press the ball in at the point where the sternum articulates with the right clavicle (figure 16.8). This inward pressure on the joint is what gives the bones of the sternum and clavicle a little space at their articulation, making it possible to move the clavicle out laterally. Extend your right arm and

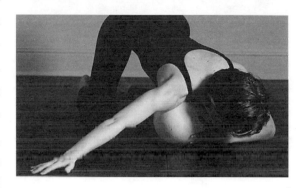

FIGURE 16.8

support yourself with the left hand on the floor. Roll laterally along the clavicle, over the origin of the clavicular head of the pectoralis major and out to its insertion.

As you roll out along the clavicle, you are also releasing the subclavius muscle, which originates at the first rib and inserts at the inferior shaft of the clavicle, as well as the insertion of the pectoralis minor muscle at the coracoid process of the scapula.

Repeat on the other side.

Side-of-the-Rib-Cage Routine

Begin with the basic side routine, rolling up from the hip (see chapter 6). When the ball is between the hip and the lower margin of the ribs, wait and breathe. After you roll above the floating ribs, make sure you are truly lying on your side, not tilting toward your front or back. Stay and breathe here, then roll slightly to the back (figure 16.9). Lean back onto the ball and breathe.

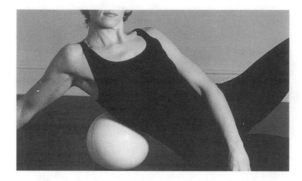

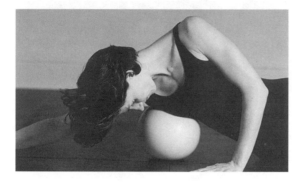

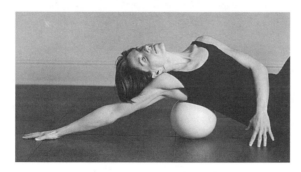

Now roll the ball toward the spine, breathing into the ribs underneath it. Roll to the side again and then to the front of the body, as far as you comfortably can (figure 16.10), and breathe. This is a tight area, and most people feel extremely vulnerable rolling the ball in toward the heart. Tell your clients that this part of the routine will not be easy, and they may want to take some of their weight off the ball and onto their arms and legs. Roll as far toward the sternum as you can; men will be able to roll farther than most women. Roll the ball back to the side and then a couple of ribs higher.

Again begin to breathe, visualizing that you are softening the rib cage and the intercostal muscles, letting the ball sink in deeper. When you feel the ribs and intercostals starting to release, begin rolling back toward the spine (figure 16.11). Your head is resting on your shoulder and your right arm should be extended as far out on the floor as possible. Make sure your breath moves fully and equally into your front, side, and back. As you roll toward the spine you cross the origin of the latissimus dorsi muscle at the lower three ribs and the inferior angle of the scapula. This movement actually peels the muscle away from the ribs. You are also crossing the muscle fibers of the trapezius, releasing any hold it might have on the ribs between T12 and T6. Now roll back to the side, and then over to the front.

The ball will now be in the area of breast tissue, so women must work very gently. Because breast tissue is softer than muscle and contains structures that can be injured, you should never roll over the breast tissue. However, you can lift the breast and try to roll underneath it. In fact, separating the breast tissue from the ribs and muscles is quite important. Women generally do not think about what lies under the breast tissue, and they tend to believe that they cannot move their breasts around. As a result, the breast tissue becomes attached to muscle and rib and therefore cannot move or breathe. However, the more circulation you can direct into that area, the healthier the breast tissue will be. Keeping breasts free and mobile will decrease congestion and breast sensitivity, especially premenstrual tenderness. While a practitioner cannot lift a client's breast tissue to stimulate the tissues underneath, a woman can do it for herself.

Closer to the underarm the pressure exerted by the ball will be more painful and the ribs and intercostals will take longer to soften, so wait and push your breath into your side a bit longer before moving to the back. As you roll to the back you are moving toward the lateral border of the scapula, from the inferior angle to the axilla, and releasing the anterior serratus muscle, which means that this time you are pushing the scapula toward the spine.

Since you cannot roll directly over the ribs here, roll onto the scapula. The weight of your body and the pressure of the ball on the scapula, in conjunction with your breathing, will allow you to stimulate the ribs under the scapula. The inhalation will expand those ribs, so you will also be releasing the ribs from the inside out. Without rolling all the way to the spine, roll off the scapula back onto your side, then toward the front.

As you roll anteriorly, crossing the tendons of the pectoralis major and minor muscles, the tissue is much tighter. With the ball in the axilla, wait and breathe, sinking the ball as far in toward the first three ribs as you can, your weight angled more toward the chest (figure 16.12). Feel the ball pushing into the anterior ribs rather than the armpit. As you breathe, try to sink into those first three ribs a little more with each exhalation.

Now lift your hips, using your left hand to balance so that the additional weight goes directly into the first three

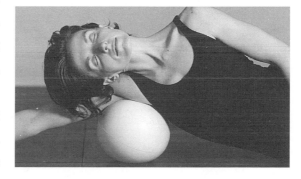

FIGURE 16.12

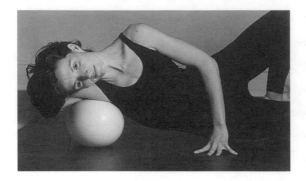

FIGURE 16.13

ribs (figure 16.13). Breathe, trying to soften the ribs. See if you can begin to roll the ball anteroinferiorly, pushing it against those first three ribs. The goal is a downward movement of the whole rib cage—releasing the first three ribs is essential for achieving this.

To get a clear sense of the importance of releasing the rib cage, lie on the floor for a few moments, then get up and walk around, noticing which parts of your body have been affected by this routine. Look at your hips, shoulders, arms, and face, and check your breathing, observing the lateral movement of your ribs in the mirror as you breathe. What changes do you notice?

Repeat this routine on the left side.

17

PREGNANCY
AND
POSTPARTUM

This chapter gives adaptations of previous routines that will prevent or relieve problems during pregnancy and the postpartum period.

Pregnancy

From the moment a woman conceives, her body begins to change as its structure adapts to accommodate the pregnancy. The abdominal muscles in the pubic region tighten as the pelvic area contracts to protect the fetus. As the fetus develops, pressure into the pubic area intensifies. Because the weight increases slowly, in most cases the pelvis can adapt to it. However, most of us have some form of pelvic distortion that we developed early in life. This distortion will manifest clinically either during pregnancy or postpartum.

As more weight bears down into the pelvis, a woman's posture shifts. Some women bend forward into the additional weight; others compensate by leaning backward and turning their feet out when they walk. Another common problem created by pregnancy weight is pain in the legs. Women develop cramps, swelling, varicosities, and general tiredness and heaviness in the legs. In addition, increased breast size can cause shoulder problems and collapse of the thoracic cage.

The most important preventive practice during pregnancy is keeping the spine and torso as long, flexible, strong, and erect as possible to minimize the amount of pressure affecting the pelvic area. The second most important practice is maintaining maximum range of motion in the legs and keeping them released from the hips so they will not suffer from the extra weight or develop restrictions or circulatory problems. If the pregnancy is exacerbating a hip imbalance, leg routines along with maintaining length in the spine will help correct hip misalignment and insure proper pelvis alignment, thus minimizing discomfort.

Women are told to keep their abdominal muscles strong during pregnancy. However, as I said in chapter 9, strong muscles are long and toned. Maintaining such muscles will provide as much space and support as possible for the fetus and internal organs. And the longer and more open the abdominal area remains during pregnancy, the sooner the abdominal muscles will regain their original tone after delivery.

Routines for Pregnancy

● BASIC BACK AND SIDE ROUTINES

Daily rolling up both sides of the body (figures 17.1 and 17.2), up both sides of the spine, and up the center of the spine (figures 17.3, 17.4, and 17.5) will keep the spine long and strong. Since many people find it difficult to stay directly on their side and tend to roll anteriorly, make sure women understand that they should *never* allow the ball to press into the abdomen. It is generally safe to tell pregnant women to keep the ball slightly to the back, with the front of the body tilted toward the ceiling. The basic side routine will maintain balance between the front and back

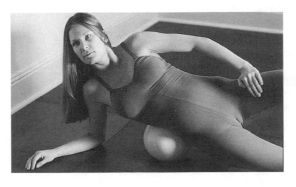

FIGURE 17.1

of the torso and prevent the shoulders from dropping forward in response to the additional weight.

LOWER BACK VARIATIONS

The first lower back routine described in chapter 8 will effectively maintain maximum length in the abdomen and help relieve lower back discomfort by stretching out the quadratus lumborum and lower latissimus dorsi. As you raise your legs, keep your bent knees separated to avoid putting pressure into the abdomen, and breathe into the lower back. Visualize your breath filling and expanding the whole lower back. Then lower the feet to the ground using the abdominal muscles; the more slowly you do this movement, the more effective it is. This movement strengthens the lower abdominal muscles.

Slowly slide the feet out on the floor, extending the legs to their maximum; the further forward you stretch them, the longer the abdominals become. Breathe in this position, concentrating on stretching the belly out during the inhalation and relaxing on the exhalation. Visualize with each inhalation that you are providing space for the fetus to stretch out into. This exercise takes the weight off your legs and anterior pelvis and also lets you

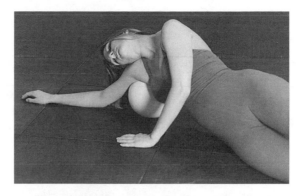

FIGURE 17.2

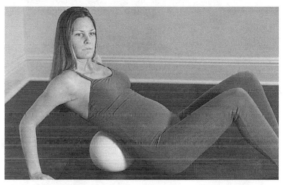

FIGURE 17.3

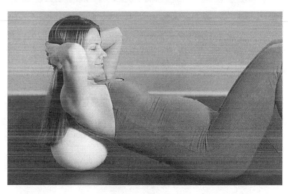

FIGURE 17.4

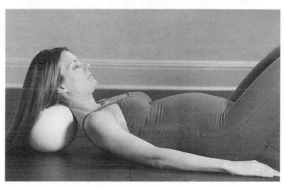

FIGURE 17.5

feel the quadriceps elongating downward as the abdominal muscles elongate upward.

You can also do some leg exercises in this position. Raise one leg straight up toward the ceiling while stretching the other leg along the floor, then reverse the legs. Extending the legs upward takes pressure off them, increasing circulation; raising and lowering the legs also strengthens the lower abdominals. Begin with ten to fifteen leg lifts and slowly work up to fifty.

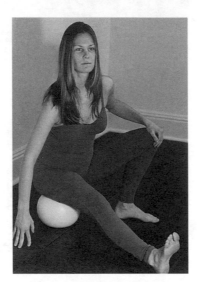

FIGURE 17.6

LEG ROUTINES

The leg routines in chapter 10 are extremely beneficial throughout pregnancy to maintain maximum circulation and range of motion. If time is short, you can do the routines for the hamstrings (figure 17.6), quadriceps (figure 17.7), and adductors (figure 17.8) two to three times a week. It is not necessary to work all the way to the feet at each session; you can stop at the insertions of these muscles at the knee. The most important factor is to keep the connection between the pelvis and femur unrestricted. Include five minutes of rolling the bottoms of the feet to help prevent tiredness, cramping, and fluid retention.

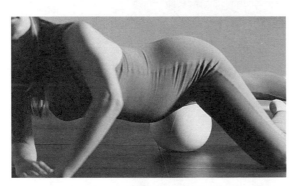

FIGURE 17.7

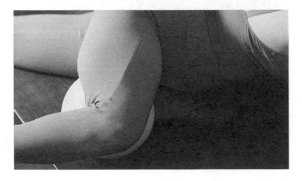

FIGURE 17.8

Postpartum

During pregnancy the body adjusts to the fetus. The intestines are pushed up and to the sides and there is extra pressure on the bladder; the other organs also accommodate the growing fetus. After labor and delivery the fetus is suddenly gone. The internal organs remain displaced around an empty area in the center of the abdomen and the abdominal muscles that were stretching for nine months have nothing to hold anymore.

During delivery the pelvic ligaments, softened by hormones, allow the baby to pass through the pelvis. The body is left traumatized, having lost much of its muscle memory and its proper alignment. Labor and delivery have tremendous impact on a woman's body. No matter how much exercise she has done, she has never inflicted that much pressure and trauma on her pelvis.

Any imbalance or weakness present before delivery is made worse by the intense pressure bearing down on the pelvis during delivery. For example, in all of us one leg is stronger than the other. During delivery, when the woman uses her legs to push, this imbalance can cause a structural shift in the pelvis as well as a state of contraction persisting after delivery, due to intense strain of the adductors. Similarly, many women have a disposition to back problems that does not manifest clinically until they have a child. If you ask women with children who come to you with a back problem when their first symptoms occurred, 95 percent of them will say they never had a back problem before they had their first child.

Left after delivery with a weak body and unstable pelvis, the new mother now has a baby to take care of. Like all mothers, she lifts the baby, puts it down, and carries it more on one side than the other. This imbalance imposes extra stress on already weak, strained muscles.

Moreover, the hormone that stimulates milk secretion during breastfeeding also contracts the uterus, which in turn contracts all the surrounding tissues. Accordingly, many women complain that their pelvis is tight when they wake up in the morning. The combination of internal contraction, externally weak muscles, and strained ligaments leaves new mothers vulnerable to injury—trying to lift something with no abdominal support is a perfect way to strain your back.

Women have never been given adequate education about the importance of checking the alignment of the pelvis right after childbirth, or about how to relieve the shock and trauma the body has undergone. Although there are many pregnancy and postpartum exercise classes available, those classes do not teach women how to study their postpartum alignment to determine what structural problems need to be addressed *before* they begin to exercise. Simply strengthening the abdominals, which is what these classes tend to focus on, will not correct a pelvic problem.

Postpartum Routines

Postpartum work begins with the basic routines for back, sides, and front, along with variations, to restore optimal upright posture (see chapters 5–7). Women who have had caesarean sections should wait at least eight weeks to put any pressure into the abdomen, or until the physician gives them approval.

BASIC BACK AND SIDE ROUTINES

Over nine months of carrying extra weight, the spine is pulled downward. It is therefore extremely important to elongate the torso after childbirth. As you do these routines, imagine you are elongating your muscles up from the pelvis, restoring length and tone. In addition, visualize that you are lifting your vertebrae, repositioning them one at a time to restore intervertebral space and bring the spine to an upright position, with energy flowing more freely upward.

FRONT ROUTINE AND VARIATIONS

Visualize the ball lifting your abdominal muscles while doing the basic front routine. You will also be lifting your intestines and bladder, restoring them to their normal positions. (The information in chapter 9 on correcting prolapses will also be of use to you here.)

Do not mindlessly go through the motions of this routine. You are rebuilding your body and restoring abdominal tone to support your internal organs—see this process as you do the routine, keeping your intention crystal clear. Visualize each muscle strand lifting and being charged with new energy. This will bring length, tone, and vitality to all the muscle fibers.

Continue to practice the basic abdominal routine for at least one month. As your muscles become more toned, add the following variation, which is even more effective for restoring true length in the muscle fibers.

Instead of lying flat over the ball, raise yourself up on your hands, as in the cobra pose from yoga (figure 17.9). Slowly roll

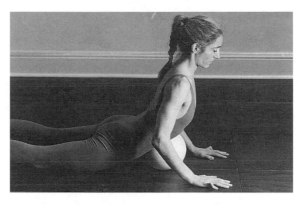

FIGURE 17.9

upward, breathing at each point, feeling the muscles being stimulated to elongate. Work up to the point just below the ribs. The ball pushes the abdominal muscles up as you roll, lifting the internal organs. Since in this position the ball sinks more deeply into the abdomen, it also begins to elongate the psoas major together with the more superficial abdominal muscles. At the same time, the release of the psoas major protects the lower back by relieving tension in the anterior lumbar spine.

Because the next variation requires more abdominal strength, it may be eight weeks or so before you are ready for it. This variation should be practiced in the same session as the previous routine.

Place the ball partly on the pubic bone but mostly in the pelvic area. Stretch your arms above your head and stretch your legs long behind you. Keeping the knees bent and together, slowly lift both legs on an inhalation (figure 17.10), then exhale and lower them. As you lift on the inhalation, you draw air into the lungs. With this air still inside you, pull your abdominal muscles in toward the spine and upward. This tightens the muscle fibers of the lower abdomen. Hold for ten seconds, then exhale.

The first lower back routine in chapter 8 is also good for strengthening the abdominals after delivery. Raising and lowering the legs increases abdominal

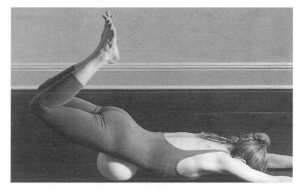

FIGURE 17.10

strength and elongates the lower back muscles. When the legs are extended out on the floor, be sure that you work to elongate them out from the pelvis, while also visualizing that you are elongating the abdominal muscles up from the pelvis.

LEG ROUTINES

Following delivery there is likely to be pressure and heaviness in the legs because of the extra weight they have carried. To relieve the legs as well as to break any misalignment pattern in the hip that might have developed while carrying the additional weight, do the leg routines in chapter 10 to recover stability, strength, and increased circulation. Focus particularly on the adductors, because these muscles take the most strain during pregnancy and labor.

Rolling the bottoms of the feet for five minutes is effective now too, to prevent tiredness and cramping and to begin increasing circulation upward from the extremities.

THE
EFFECTS
OF AGING

All of us will be getting older, but we do not need to accept the structural restrictions that most people take for granted as part of the aging process.

In terms of the musculoskeletal system, the aging process involves a slow collapsing of the body. As gravity takes over, muscle tone and mass are lost, the muscles contract and shorten, the abdomen drops into the pelvis, the extra weight from the abdomen exerts an additional downward pull and causes a general slowing of metabolism, and arthritis and circulatory problems set in. Women are likely to notice much earlier in life than men such effects of decreased circulation as varicosities, cold extremities, and a general tendency to feel cold more easily.

Many people go through life without noticing these changes until one day they realize that an activity that was once easy now tires them out, or that their range of motion limits their performance in a sport they used to excel at. It is at such moments that you hear the remark, "I must be getting old." Such comments signal an acceptance of the aging process that is characteristic of our culture.

Similarly, when younger people who have a structural injury are left with restricted movement, that is the beginning of the aging process for that joint. Our culture tells us to accept this condition as inevitable. But in fact, we do not have to. If people knew that they did not have to accept such restrictions, and had access to information telling them how to restore full range of motion to their joints, they could do so.

In the same way, if older people were told how to take care of their structure they would not have to accept the restrictions on movement that our culture sees as inherent in the aging process. Our society emphasizes diet and fitness, which implies cardiovascular exercise. But this understanding of fitness does not help prevent physical limitations. In fact, in many cases it adds to them.

Restrictions to range of motion in one or many joints signal the presence of osteoarthritis, which is commonly associated with the aging process. Wear and tear causes narrowing of joints with degeneration of cartilage, and the body attempts to heal itself by depositing calcium as spurs (osteophytes) on the bones.

The effects of arthritis are particularly noticeable in people's body structure. Typically in people age sixty and above, the spine shortens and loses its backward mobility, the head drops forward, the cervical spine curves anteriorly, the rib cage narrows inward, the shoulders droop, and the arms hang forward. The limbs move in walking but the spine does not move with them. The narrowing of the chest causes the abdomen to protrude, which not only puts pressure on the lower back but also weakens the abdominal muscles. Weak abdominals put more pressure in the anterior pelvis, which in turn restricts the quadriceps, limiting leg movement.

When the spine collapses it loses flexibility and intervertebral space, and circulation to the vertebrae decreases. Because the skeletal structure is bearing weight downward, the bones and intervertebral disks become subject to greater pressure and wear away more rapidly, which contributes to the shrinking process and the formation of osteophytes. If, on the other hand, the spine remains upright, the muscles will have their full length and function from origin to insertion, the vertebrae will receive much more circulation, and the spine will remain elastic.

Studies have found that the one part of the body in which we can control the aging process is muscle development. If, therefore, we consciously keep our muscles toned, alive, and taking their full length throughout life, we will be able to maintain healthy muscle fiber that gives joints optimal range of motion. As muscle contraction and tightness release, circulation improves, and this in turn improves bone quality.

In counteracting the aging process, Body Rolling works on bone as well as muscle. As I have explained, putting direct pressure on bone and waiting at each point stimulates circulation to that bone and also stimulates response in any muscle with any attachments on that bone. By waking the bone, therefore, you also awaken muscle fiber.

Much concern has been focused recently on osteoporosis in postmenopausal women. In this condition the quality of bone changes—due to diminished circulation, the bone tissue receives fewer nutrients. In addition, since the hormonal condition at menopause inhibits calcium intake, calcium is leached from bone. As a result, bones lose density and grow increasingly brittle.

Studies have found that, by stimulating bone, weight-bearing exercise can prevent and possibly reverse osteoporosis. Weight-bearing is nothing more than pressure exerted on bone. Body Rolling is actually a mild form of weight-bearing exercise in which the pressure is never more than the person's own body weight. Too much weight can damage a bone, but using Body Rolling to limit and control the amount of weight placed on bone is an ideal way for elderly people to stimulate healthy bone. My clinical experience has been that, when women diagnosed with osteoporosis directly stimulate bone by rolling on the ball, their bone becomes less brittle and more flexible.

In working with older people, it is essential to evaluate their muscle quality, circulation, and bone quality before beginning ball work. As a rule, older people are less flexible and therefore need to work with a softer ball. You can evaluate bone quality by having the client lie on several types of balls to feel which one provides the most comfortable pressure. The wrong type of ball will cause pain or discomfort, an adequate indication that the client's bone is too rigid for that ball.

Since the rib cage is the part of the body that can break most easily, older people should not initially do Body Rolling in this area. The rib cage should be the last part of the body they work with, and they should work with the greatest caution there.

All the routines given in previous chapters can be adapted to whatever the client's range of motion and general health and strength dictate. If someone uses a walker, for example, look for what part of the body retains the greatest range of motion. Have the client begin there; as she achieves freer movement, you will see the body virtually unwind itself and demonstrate where it is next willing to increase its range of motion.

Suppose the person has a restricted neck. As the neck begins to release, she may become aware of tension in the shoulder and want that to be released to go with her newly mobile neck. You might then suggest a modified side routine.

You can also look closely to see where gaining greater flexibility would really make a difference in someone's quality of life. For example, most older people are amazed when, after receiving some hands-on bodywork and practicing the ball routines, they find they can turn their neck twenty degrees more in either direction than they have for ten years. With this added mobility and freedom, they receive a whole new lease on life.

The following routines cover elderly people who are mobile and active and also those confined to a bed or chair. The routines for the bed- and chair-ridden are also excellent for people of any age who are paralyzed, recovering from a stroke, or bedridden after surgery. Body Rolling can prevent phlebitis and other circulatory problems, as well as general stiffness from immobility. These routines are also great to practice on airplanes.

Routines for Mobile, Active People

Use a soft ball that has a lot of give when weight is placed on it. The following routines are for the parts of the body that people need most for mobility: the spine and the legs. Any person who can get around can safely begin a Body Rolling practice by working the spine and the back of the legs.

Keeping the spine healthy and flexible is the key to slowing down the aging process. Have clients begin with the basic back routine, working up each side of the spine for a couple of weeks before working up the center (see chapter 5). Working up the side of the spine stimulates more bone, tendon, and muscle than does working up the center, where the ball is only on the spinous processes. Going up the sides also stimulates the larger external back muscles, which must be released before you can release the erector spinae muscles.

At the same time you can give clients the basic routine for the back of the leg (see chapter 10). Beginning at the posterior iliac crest to release the gluteus maximus, they can roll down toward its insertion, then to the ischium. Have them sit a few moments and roll around on the ischium. Most elderly people will not have the flexibility to lean forward, so they should keep their hands behind them or at their sides. Last, they can slowly roll down the hamstrings and as far down to the ankle as possible.

These two exercises do not require much strength. For the quadriceps routine, however, people must support themselves on their arms, and some people will not have enough strength to do this. But if they can raise themselves up on their elbows without hurting their neck or shoulders, you can also give them the quadriceps routine.

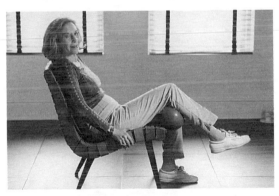

FIGURE 18.1

Routines for People in Chairs

Use a six-inch ball for these routines. Do them in the order presented here.

To work the legs, place the ball under one thigh, as close to the ischium as possible. Sit on the ball for a few moments, then slowly roll the ball toward the edge of the chair until it is pressing into both the back of the knee and the thigh (figure 18.1). Then roll it just over the edge of the chair so that the ball presses into the knee and the top of the calf (figure 18.2). (For this you need a chair with a front side that the ball can press against.)

To stimulate the quadriceps, place the ball in the crease of the hip and lean on it with your elbow or forearm (figure 18.3).

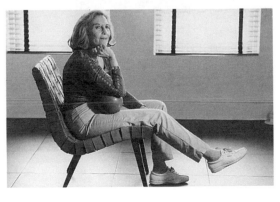

FIGURE 18.2

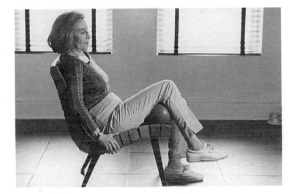

FIGURE 18.3

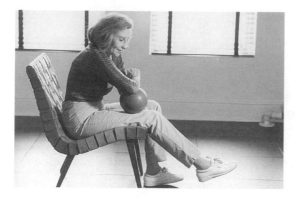

FIGURE 18.4

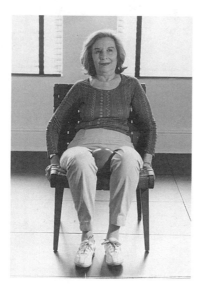

FIGURE 18.5

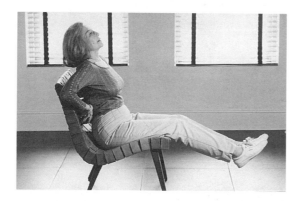

FIGURE 18.6

Roll down the thigh as close to the knee as possible, at each point pressing into the ball with the elbow or forearm (figure 18.4).

Next, work the adductors. Put the ball between your thighs (figure 18.5), squeeze, and let go. Work this way down to the knees.

Work up each side of the spine by putting the ball between the base of your spine and the back of the chair and then using your hands to move it up point by point (figure 18.6) and leaning back against it (figure 18.7). (You may need assistance for this.)

To do a front routine, put the ball at the pubic bone and push it with your hands gently into the belly (figure 18.8). Roll the ball up from the belly, breathing at each point. At the sternum, push the ball in gently at each point, pushing the breath out against the ball (figure 18.9). This action lifts the sternum, helping you sit more erectly.

To work the sides, hold the ball under your arm and sit straight (figure 18.10), breathing out into the side of the rib cage for three minutes on each side. This routine helps open the shoulder and increases the oxygen supply into the chest, shoulder, and head.

Routines for People in Bed

People who are bedridden easily develop circulatory problems, which lead to infections in the toes or feet. Rolling down the backs of the legs and up the spine is wonderful for keeping the circulation moving and reducing the chance of developing bed-sores or gangrene.

Most bedridden people will need assistance for the following routines, so you should teach them to the person's primary caretaker. Explain that the person doing the rolling should apply only as much pressure as the bedridden person feels to be pleasurable; there should be no discomfort associated with this exercise.

To work the legs of people lying on the back, place the ball underneath the leg and hold it at each point from thigh to ankle. Next, roll the ball down the quadriceps medially, centrally, and laterally, then down to the foot.

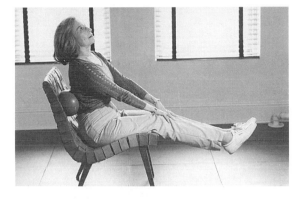

FIGURE 18.7

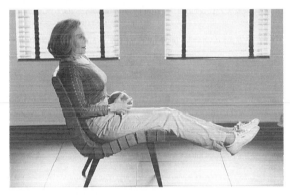

FIGURE 18.8

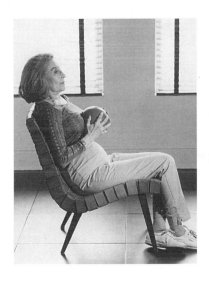

FIGURE 18.9

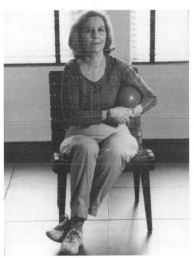

FIGURE 18.10

If the client can lie face down, you or the caretaker can gently do the back routine for him or her, rolling the ball up from the sacrum. At each point the client should breathe into the ball. Roll as far up the neck as possible. Finally, roll down the back from the neck on each side.

People who can move around in bed may try lying on the ball and rolling up each side of the spine themselves.

CONCLUSION
An Open-Ended Practice

My hope for this book is that you will find in it new techniques and insights that you can integrate into your existing body-therapy practice. Even more important, I hope that you will now have tools to keep your own body healthy and pain free.

Once body therapists have learned anatomy in their professional training, they often forget the details. Body Rolling is a wonderful tool for continuously reviewing your own anatomy, sensing and exploring specific muscles and learning the connections among them. You will find that the body can also be a kind of research laboratory for exploring a wider range of possible factors that may be involved when you are treating specific conditions in clients.

I urge you to find time in your sessions with clients to become more an educator than a fixer, teaching the routines presented here as educational tools they can use at home. By giving a client an intellectual understanding of what muscle connections are involved in her problem, you give her a way of thinking about it and responding to it herself, instead of simply taking it to you to fix. In this way she will feel more a part of her own healing process and more in control of it.

Beyond these practical benefits, however, Body Rolling will help both you and your clients develop kinesthetic awareness. From childhood our minds are trained cognitively in audio, visual, and verbal skills, while our bodies are sent to gym class and sports programs, where we learn to exercise but not to feel what happens in the body while we exercise. As adults, therefore, we lack the ability to perceive our body signals and use them along with our thinking and intuition to process information. Although many people practice some kind of fitness activity, they are not necessarily listening to the body while they do it, so they may miss any warning signals the body sends.

People who become body-therapy practitioners often maintain this split between mind and body: they use the mind to analyze what is happening in the client's body while their hands simply take orders to perform a given physical technique. Even people who have "great hands" might be unaware of what is happening in another person's body because they cannot read that body's response to their touch.

Because people do not learn kinesthetic awareness during their traditional education, it needs to be specifically taught. Body Rolling will educate both you and your clients to develop a keen ability to feel changes in the body.

Increasing your kinesthetic awareness has an additional, far deeper potential. Every life experience is embedded somewhere in the body. Body Rolling can lead to open-ended self-explorations in which you work through layer after layer, freeing muscular and energetic blockages. The deep sink becomes endless; and Body Rolling becomes a profound form of meditation—stilling, relaxing, leading toward self-realization.

RESOURCES

BODY LOGIC AND BODY ROLLING PROGRAMS

Body Logic offers training programs for bodywork and fitness professionals that cover the more specialized applications of Body Rolling. Body Rolling classes for lay people are also available. Information on these programs, on Body Logic workshops and certification training, and on individual Body Logic sessions is available from the Body Logic studio.

Call or write: Body Logic

295 West 11th Street, Suite 1F

New York, NY 10014

1-800-877-8429

You can also reach Body Logic by e-mail at yamunazake@aol.com or on the World Wide Web at http://www.bodylogic.com.

PURCHASING BALLS

Specialized balls for Body Rolling are available by mail order. Call or write for a catalog.

EDUCATIONAL REFERENCES

I strongly recommend that you have good anatomical illustrations at hand as you practice the ball work. These aids make visualizing the muscles much easier, which deepens somatic experience, especially when you are working on your own. Suggested references are:

Blandine Calais-Germain, *Anatomy of Movement* (Seattle: Eastland Press, 1993). Recommended for its excellent descriptions and illustrations of each muscle's range of movement.

Kay W. Sieg and Sandra P. Adams, *Illustrated Essentials of Musculoskeletal Anatomy*, 2d ed. (Gainesville: Megabooks, 1985). Large, clear diagrams of each muscle.

Flash Anatomy, *The Muscles* (flash cards), 2d ed. (Anaheim: Flash Anatomy Inc., 1989). These clearly drawn diagrams are extremely useful—line up the cards on the floor for all the muscles you intend to work.

ACKNOWLEDGMENTS

Above all, I thank my parents for always believing in my capabilities, which gave me the confidence to strike out on my own path.

I am grateful to Swami Vishnudevananda and the Sivananda organization for giving me yoga as a physical discipline when I was fourteen.

Thanks also to my daughter Yael. It was her birth that inspired the development of this work.

Special thanks to Esther Lampert, who worked beside me throughout the birth and growth of Body Logic.

Thank you to Stephanie Golden for agreeing to do this project with me and for her incredible patience and professionalism (and to Stephan Bodian, former editor of *Yoga Journal*, for originally putting us together).

I thank Dr. Jose Luis Palazzi for his belief in and support of Body Logic, and for hours of discussion on the body's structure.

Much thanks to Susan Davidson, our editor at Healing Arts Press, whose knowledge of the body and belief in the Body Rolling work played a major role in bringing this book to fruition.

Tim Geaney's understanding of the work enabled him to capture the movement and sensation of each routine in his exquisite photographs—thank you.

I am grateful to Susan Marchand, Patty Jordan, and Sandra Leatherford for modeling some of the routines.

Thank you to Jonathan Paskow, for learning patience with me.

Finally, thanks to my clients and students who have believed in me and supported my work. I have learned almost everything I know today about the body from all of you.

INDEX

Rolfing

*Reestablishing the natural alignment and structural integration
of the human body for vitality and well-being*

Ida P. Rolf, Ph.D.

ISBN 0-89281-335-0 • $24.95 pb

304 pages, 8 x 10 • 600 black-and-white illustrations

This seminal work made its debut to critical acclaim in 1977, and has remained the most important reference for Rolfers around the world. In this new edition of the original and classic text, Dr. Rolf illustrates her theory and practice of Structural Integration.

Developed by Dr. Rolf, Structural Integration—Rolfing— aligns and balances the physical body within its gravitational field, through systematic manipulation of the connective tissue that surrounds the muscles. Rolfing has helped thousands of people to stand taller, look better, move with greater ease, and have a greater sense of vitality and well-being.

"In the case of humans, structure and function are meaningless, one without the other; so that when Ida Rolf integrates structure, as nobody else can, she improves functioning. Rolfing was a revealing and unforgettable experience for me." **Moshe Feldenkrais**

Rolfing and Physical Reality

Ida P. Rolf, Ph.D.

Edited and with an introduction by Rosemary Feitis

ISBN 0-89281-380-6 • $14.95 pb

215 pages, 5 3/8 x 8 1/4

Rolf's inspired work has delivered millions from the damages of age and injury on the body. Now one of her foremost students edits a long-awaited companion work to Rolf's earlier scholarly work, *Rolfing*.

Just as enlightening in a different way, the current work captures the more intimate experiences and recollections of a remarkable healer—Rolf's thoughts, insights, and intuitions are presented in short snippets. We come to understand the extraordinary mind and heart behind the scientist in her own reflections on her work.

"In her earlier writing, Dr. Rolf's formal training was at the forefront. This intriguing work captures the dazzling immediacy of her personality." **The Book Reader**

"…a perceptive and affectionate introduction to Ida Rolf and her therapeutic system. One is treated to selections from Rolf's intuitive, intelligent, and humorous commentaries on the background, philosophy, and technique of Rolfing." **Library Journal**

Balancing Your Body

A Self-help Approach to Rolfing Movement

Mary Bond
ISBN 0-89281-642-2 • $14.95 pb
224 pages, 6 x 9

Rolfing Movement goes beyond good posture and movement efficiency. It combines touch and verbal messages to help you become more responsive to your body's inner cues. By responding appropriately to these internal messages, you create new freedom in your physical expression, which leads to a noticeable increase in health and vitality.

Mary Bond holds a master's degree in dance from UCLA and trained with Dr. Ida Rolf. She is a certified Rolfer and Rolfing Movement teacher.

"Meticulous instructions for exploring how you hold and move every part of your body. The rewards aren't to be underestimated. Rolfing Movement goes to the core of why people feel stiff and disjointed."
Natural Health

Balancing Your Body (audiocassette)

A Self-Help Approach to Rolfing Movement

Mary Bond
ISBN 0-89281-643-0 • $10.95 one 90-minute audiocassette

This recording is the ideal companion to *Balancing Your Body*. Here, the author guides you through a series of structural awareness explorations based on those in the book. You will learn to recognize and respond in appropriate ways to the body's inner messages, find new freedom in your physical expression, and improve your well-being and vitality.

The Body of Life

Creating New Pathways for Sensory Awareness and Fluid Movement

Thomas Hanna
ISBN 0-89281-481-0 • $12.95 pb
224 pages, 5 3/8 x 8 1/4

In this classic book on bodywork education, Thomas Hanna builds on the theories of Functional Integration, a method that applies gentle physical manipulation to fine-tune the nervous system and eliminate involuntary responses of tension, anxiety, and emotional pain. Through case histories, the author describes methods for improving bodily coordination, balance, and range of movement. He also surveys the pioneering work of Moshe Feldenkrais, who devised the system of Functional Integration, and many other somatic educators. Hanna's engaging account offers a profound understanding of the precise relationship between mind and body that can be applied in day-to-day living.

The Reflexology Manual

An Easy-to-Use Illustrated Guide to the Healing Zones of the Hands and Feet

Pauline Wills

ISBN 0-89281-547-7 • $19.95 pb

144 pages, 8 1/2 x 11

150 color photographs and illustrations

An ancient therapy used in China, Egypt, and India, reflexology provides effective treatment for many disorders. Reflexology harnesses the body's healing energy by stimulating specific pressure points on the hands and feet, alleviating the energy blocks that can cause pain or disability and restoring optimum health. In *The Reflexology Manual*, the practical text guides you in mastering these self-help techniques, and color photographs illustrate a full reflexology treatment step by step. Ideal for beginners as well as experienced students.

Ayurvedic Massage

Traditional Indian Techniques for Balancing Body and Mind

Harish Johari

ISBN 0-89281-489-6 • $19.95 pb

160 pages, 8 1/2 x 11

115 black-and-white illustrations

Ayurvedic Massage is based on one of the oldest systems of medicine in the world, and yet is the first new massage therapy introduced to the West since shiatsu. Ayurvedic massage concentrates on the *marmas*, subtle energy points that respond to gentle manipulation. It works on both the physical and mental levels, enabling the body to repair and renew itself.

Soft-Tissue Manipulation

A Practitioner's Guide to the Diagnosis and Treatment of
Soft-Tissue Dysfunction and Reflex Activity

Leon Chaitow, N.D., D.O.

ISBN 0-89281-276-1 • $49.95 cloth

144 pages, 7 1/2 x 10

70 two-color illustrations

This authoritative textbook provides a working knowledge of neuro-muscular technique, a diagnostic and treatment method for restoring the structural, functional, and postural integrity of the body.

"Chaitow is a visionary in bringing together different alternative and complementary health systems and points of view into a form that offers new therapeutic possibilities."

Robert King, President
American Massage Therapy Association

Amma Therapy

A Complete Textbook of Oriental Bodywork and Medical Principles

Tina Sohn and Robert Sohn
ISBN 0-89281-488-8 • $45.00 cloth
448 pages, 8 1/2 x 11
170 black-and-white illustrations

From the founders of the Wholistic Health Center in Manhasset, New York comes Amma Therapy—a groundbreaking form of bodywork that incorporates elements of acupuncture, herbalism, diet, and exercise to restore, promote, and maintain the movement of Qi (life energy) within the body. This profusely illustrated guide takes you step-by-step through the entire Amma Therapy treatment, and provides diagnosis and protocols for many common conditions.

BodyWork Shiatsu

Bringing the Art of Finger Pressure to the Massage Table

Carl Dubitsky
ISBN 0-89281-526-4 • $24.95 pb
256 pages, 8 1/2 x 11
275 black-and-white illustrations

The director of Healthsprings Clinic in Boulder, Colorado presents his innovative method for integrating the energetic concepts and techniques of shiatsu with Western osteopathic and therapeutic massage. His analysis of the muscular anatomy of the traditional energetic points and pathways provides a new perspective on this ancient healing art, making shiatsu techniques more accessible and comprehensible to health professionals and body workers of all schools.

"A well-researched and thoughtful bridge between bodywork and modern medicine…its thoroughness and precision provide the depth of concrete information that is missing from virtually all other works."
Deane Juhan, author of *Job's Body*

Acupuncture Imaging

Perceiving the Energy Pathways of the Body

Mark D. Seem, Ph.D., Dipl. Ac. (NCCA)
ISBN 0-89281-375-X • $19.95 cloth
96 pages, 5 3/8 x 8 1/4

This accessible guide, developed as a teaching tool for practitioners of meridian therapies, enables patients to gain a better understanding of the energy pathways used in their treatment. The author shows how physical, emotional, and psychological problems can be seen in terms of disrupted energy flow, and helps the patient see, feel, and conceptualize these disturbances in a way that enables the healing process to succeed.

Acupuncture Imaging is a valuable resource for health professionals, teachers, students, and patients of all energetic and meridian therapies, including acupuncture, shiatsu, acupressure, and bodyworkers, as well as psychotherapists and others interested in Eastern concepts of medicine.

Reiki Energy Medicine

Bringing the Healing Touch into Home, Hospital, and Hospice

Libby Barnett and Maggie Chambers with Susan Davidson
ISBN 0-89281-633-3 • $12.95 pb • 152 pages, 6 x 9

Reiki Energy Medicine shows how the ancient healing art of touch therapy is joining other alternative therapies in the conventional settings of hospitals, hospices, counseling centers, emergency rooms, and intensive care units. Health care practitioners report that Reiki helps to manage pain and promote healing, and gives patients an increased ability to cope. *Reiki Energy Medicine* explains the body's energy system, and describes how Reiki can be used in a variety of settings to balance energy and create the conditions needed for healing.

The Alexander Technique

How to Use Your Body Without Stress

Wilfred Barlow, M.D.
ISBN 0-89281-385-7 • $12.95 pb • 240 pages, 6 x 9

Long before Wilhelm Reich's therapeutic work or Esalen's program of total sensory awareness, F.M. Alexander discovered, mastered, and taught the secret of successful body dynamics—how to achieve a balanced physical use of the body in movement or at rest, with the minimum amount of stress and tension. Barlow demonstrates how this technique can help you discover untapped energy, relieve tension and fatigue, and learn an entirely new way of using your body.

The Body Has Its Reasons

Self-awareness Through Conscious Movement

Therese Bertherat and Carol Bernstein
ISBN 0-89281-298-2 • $10.95 pb • 152 pages, 5 3/8 x 8 1/4

This engrossing narrative introduces movement based on a profound self-awareness that frees us from limiting attitudes about ourselves and our bodies. The authors explore the many reasons for chronic aches and pains that have no apparent cause, and show how tensions can be released and a new range of movement opened up to us.

Ways to Better Breathing

Carola Speads
ISBN 0-89281-397-0 • $12.95 pb • 128 pages, 6 3/4 x 8 1/2

A life-long teacher of breathing practices shows how the quality of our breathing determines the quality of our lives. Her flexible program of gentle exercises relieves stress and benefits all who use breath consciously, including those in the performing arts and public speaking as well as those engaged in heavy physical labor. Taking only minutes a day, these exercises bring improved health, psychological well-being, energy, and creativity.

Acupuncture Energetics

A Workbook for Diagnostics and Treatment

Mark D. Seem, Ph.D., Dipl. Ac. (NCCA) • ISBN 0-89281-435-7 • $16.95 pb • 144 pages, 5 3/8 x 8 1/2

The first educational textbook on acupuncture designed for Western students and practitioners, *Acupuncture Energetics* offers an innovative approach to diagnosis and treatment planning in acupuncture that integrates Eight-Principle and Five-Phase diagnosis. A workbook section, keyed to major texts widely used in the field, includes case studies and self-study exercises, and provides an excellent resource for those who are preparing for licensure examinations.

"While the concept of Acupuncture Energetics *breaks completely new ground, the author's simple and direct approach is in line with pure Traditional Chinese Medicine. This highly original book deserves a place in the curriculum of all schools of acupuncture."*

Royston Low, Ph. D., Dr. Ac., Past President, British Acupuncture Association

Bodymind Energetics

Toward a Dynamic Model of Health

Mark D. Seem, Ph.D., Dipl. Ac. (NCCA) • ISBN 0-89281-246-X • $18.95 pb • 258 pages, 6 x 9

Through an integration of the principles of Traditional Chinese Medicine and psychosomatics, author Mark Seem moves beyond the existing medical models to develop a new energetic paradigm of health care—one that acknowledges the spirit of the individual seeking treatment as well as the fundamental connections between energy, body, and mind.

"Mark Seem's remarkable and innovative work explores new possibilities, using acupuncture to inform psychology and modern psychosomatics to expand contemporary acupuncture practices. This dialogue will not only enrich the two participant medical systems but will also contribute to the entire field of health, medicine, and healing."

Ted Kaptchuk, Author of *The Web That Has No Weaver*

Acupressure Techniques

A Self-Help Guide

Julian Kenyon, M.D. • ISBN 0-89281-280-X • $12.95 pb • 224 pages, 5 3/8 x 8 1/4

Especially written for home use, this fully illustrated guide shows how finger and thumb pressure can be safely applied over specific acupuncture points to effectively treat a wide range of disorders, including sports injuries. Dr. Kenyon is past chairman of the British Medical Acupuncture Society.

These and other Inner Traditions/Healing Arts Press titles are available at many fine bookstores. To order directly from the publisher, please call 1-800-246-8648 or mail a check or money order for the total amount, payable to Inner Traditions, plus $3.50 shipping for the first book and $1.00 for each additional book to:

Inner Traditions
P.O. Box 388, Rochester, VT 05767
1-800-246-8648 • *Be sure to request a free catalog*
Visit our Web site at www.InnerTraditions.com